Baking

with

Splenda®

Also by JoAnna M. Lund

The Healthy Exchanges Cookbook
HELP: The Healthy Exchanges Lifetime Plan
Cooking Healthy with a Man in Mind
Cooking Healthy with the Kids in Mind
Diabetic Desserts
Make a Joyful Table
Cooking Healthy Across America
A Potful of Recipes
Another Potful of Recipes
The Open Road Cookbook
Sensational Smoothies
Hot Off the Grill: The Healthy Exchanges Electric Grilling Cookbook
Cooking Healthy with Splenda®
Cooking Healthy with a Microwave
The Diabetic's Healthy Exchanges Cookbook
The Strong Bones Healthy Exchanges Cookbook
The Arthritis Healthy Exchanges Cookbook
The Heart Smart Healthy Exchanges Cookbook
The Cancer Recovery Healthy Exchanges Cookbook
String of Pearls
Family and Friends Cookbook
JoAnna's Kitchen Miracles
When Life Hands You Lemons, Make Lemon Meringue Pie
Cooking Healthy with Soy

Baking

with

Splenda®

A HEALTHY EXCHANGES® COOKBOOK

JoAnna M. Lund

with
Barbara Alpert

A Perigee Book

THE BERKLEY PUBLISHING GROUP
Published by the Penguin Group
Penguin Group (USA) Inc.
375 Hudson Street, New York, New York 10014, USA
Penguin Group (Canada), 90 Eglinton Avenue East, Suite 700, Toronto, Ontario M4P 2Y3, Canada
(a division of Pearson Penguin Canada Inc.)
Penguin Books Ltd., 80 Strand, London WC2R 0RL, England
Penguin Group Ireland, 25 St. Stephen's Green, Dublin 2, Ireland (a division of Penguin Books Ltd.)
Penguin Group (Australia), 250 Camberwell Road, Camberwell, Victoria 3124, Australia
(a division of Pearson Australia Group Pty. Ltd.)
Penguin Books India Pvt. Ltd., 11 Community Centre, Panchsheel Park, New Delhi—110 017, India
Penguin Group (NZ), cnr. Airborne and Rosedale Roads, Albany, Auckland 1310, New Zealand
(a division of Pearson New Zealand Ltd.)
Penguin Books (South Africa) (Pty.) Ltd., 24 Sturdee Avenue, Rosebank, Johannesburg 2196, South Africa
Penguin Books Ltd., Registered Offices: 80 Strand, London WC2R 0RL, England

PRINTING HISTORY
Perigee trade paperback edition / January 2006
ISBN: 0-399-53245-5

PERIGEE is a registered trademark of Penguin Group (USA) Inc.
The "P" design is a trademark belonging to Penguin Group (USA) Inc.

This book has been cataloged by the Library of Congress

PRINTED IN THE UNITED STATES OF AMERICA

10   9   8   7   6   5   4   3   2   1

Dedication

As always, this cookbook is dedicated in loving memory to my parents, Jerome and Agnes McAndrews. My mother was considered one of the very best bakers in all of Clinton County! In fact, more than a few women paid Mom to bake cakes and such for them in their pans—so they could pass the goodies off as their own! If a community bake sale was being held in Lost Nation, Iowa, the first question always was: "What is Agnes bringing? I'll buy it before it gets here!" My father was so very proud of her baking accomplishments. In fact, he delighted in bringing her baked goods with him to the Farmall Tractor Factory in Rock Island, Illinois, so he could share them with his coworkers.

I've taken many of Mom's "secret" recipes and revised them so they not only look and taste as good as hers, they're easier to prepare—and lower in fats and sugars. But I still made sure they would pass her muster before sharing them with you! Mom was a modest person, as the poem of hers that I've chosen to share with you shows. But she had much to be proud of—not only her baking skills but her writing abilities, too. I hope you enjoy her poem as much as you enjoy my recipes.

Life's Demise

When my life's task here on Earth is over,
   and Time continues to march on,
I won't leave behind wealth or riches,
   nor possessions worth a song.
But I hope to have left many pleasant memories
   for having passed this way,
Offering deeds of kindness to others,
   and a prayer for me they will say.
My monument won't be elaborate,
   like a pyramid touching the sky.
Still, I have one so priceless and precious,
   the kind that money could never buy.
For, it is three heirs I have given the world
   for the continuation of Mankind—
My most cherished possessions—three daughters—
   I have willed to God—my gift most sublime.

—Agnes Carrington McAndrews

Acknowledgments

Truly successful baking is a fine balance between ingredients, preparation method, and a well-calibrated oven. For helping me find that balance, I want to thank:

Shirley Morrow, Rita Ahlers, Phyllis Bickford, Gina Griep, and Jean Martens—my employees. While I was under deadline for this book, each pitched in and did whatever was needed—be it typing or retyping, mixing or remixing (and don't forget washing tons of dishes), tasting and retasting, and taking samples home to their families—so I could get even more feedback on the recipes. You could say they were the flour that bound this project together.

Cliff Lund—my husband. Even though he went back to long-haul trucking, he still looked forward to the samples I saved for him to try on the weekends. He especially enjoyed taste-testing the bread and cookies. And he proudly shared samples with his fellow truckers. He was the frosting on the cake of this book, so to speak.

Barbara Alpert—my writing partner. She was busy teaching, and I was busy, too, not only with this project but also with writing my monthly food newsletters, flying off to QVC, and pursuing many other Healthy Exchanges endeavors. But we found that via the Internet, we could "connect" at whatever time was convenient for each of us. Barbara became the eggs of this project. In other words, she found a way to bind my words with hers—so the finished product is better by far.

Coleen O'Shea—my literary agent. She mentioned that it was time for me to write a cookbook on baking with Splenda, because I had discovered so many more baking "secrets" since writing *Cooking Healthy with Splenda®*. She was the sweetener that made this whole project possible—and tasty.

John Duff—my publisher and editor. I've been so fortunate to work with the same person all these years, and such a helpful person he is! John was the shortening of this project—he smoothed the way for yet another Healthy Exchanges cookbook.

God—my creator and savior. When requested to create another cookbook with a very short due date, I immediately said a prayer asking for His guidance all the way. He didn't fail me—in essence, He was the yeast that made things happen quickly. He helped me rise to the occasion.

Contents

Baking is Back—and Sweeter Than Ever!   1
A Peek into My *Baking with Splenda* Pantry   9
JoAnna's Ten Commandments of Successful Cooking   11

THE RECIPES

How to Read a Healthy Exchanges Recipe   17
Yummy Yeast Breads (with Baking Tips)   19
Marvelous Muffins, Quick Breads, and More
(with Baking Tips)   55
Creamy Cakes (with Baking Tips)   87
Charming Cookies and Bars (with Baking Tips)   121
Delectable Desserts (with Baking Tips)   157
Perfect Pies and Cheesecakes (with Baking Tips)   195
Splenda Sugar Blend for Baking Beauties (with Baking Tips)   237
Grandma JO's Baking Secrets   279
Making Healthy Exchanges Work for You   307
Index   309

Baking is Back— and Sweeter Than Ever!

"If you want sweet dreams, you've got to live a sweet life."
—Barbara Kingsolver, *Animal Dreams*

Over half a century ago, back in the 1950s, women were expected to devote themselves to being perfect wives, charming hostesses, and brilliant bakers . . . and all this at a time before so many of the kitchen conveniences we now depend on were invented!

Back then, women baked elaborate cakes for family birthdays, tried to outdo one another at bake sales, and struggled to keep their figures by squeezing themselves into girdles (remember, this was before sugar substitutes were widely available!).

That was *then*, and this is now.

Then, baking was common, but so was the need to often deny ourselves the sweets we adored.

Now, after years during which baking took a backseat, lots of women—and plenty of men—are heading back to the kitchen, armed with wonderful appliances (like bread-machines!) and the culinary gift of Splenda. This healthy and delicious sugar substitute offers everyone the chance to enjoy homemade baked goods. And we no longer have to sacrifice good health or fear for our figures. Best of all, using Splenda to sweeten our goodies doesn't mean giving up good taste!

Why We Come Back to Baking

So what is it about baking that so many of us love? What draws us back to the kitchen year after year, to stir up recipes old and new?

I have a few good answers to those questions and some others.

Pull up a chair and let's visit for a while about the role that baking has played in my life and may play in yours!

Ever since the first person mixed together a little of this and that and set it to bake over a fire, baking has had a kind of magic to it, as well as a wonderful ritual. You gather your ingredients, you prepare your pans, you confer with wise and experienced cooks (in person or by using a recipe), you measure and mix and stir and pour. Then you wait and watch, entranced and intrigued, as your dough or batter is transformed by heat and time into something brand-new—something that didn't exist before but that you have somehow magically brought into the world!

Just think of that moment when the timer rings and you open the oven door. A delicious aroma emerges from the tray of cookies or muffin tin; melted chocolate oozes, the scent of cinnamon fills your kitchen, and you actually feel yourself begin to smile. What a sense of satisfaction comes over you as you place your cake pans on a cooling rack and imagine how your finished cake will look, iced and decorated. It's only a step from there to envisioning how you are going to feel when you carry your creation to the table—and your family or friends are simply dazzled!

Tradition—and the Ancient Art of Baking

I come from a long line of bakers on both sides. From my Bohemian ancestors came wonderful recipes for fruit-filled pastries that my children have adored all their lives, and from my Irish forebears I carry on the tradition of savory and hearty breads that sustain life even in tough times.

As a child, I learned about the miracle of yeast and the marvels of shortening and sugar at my mother's side. She was an artist in the kitchen and taught me to enjoy the rituals of baking—the skillful slicing of ripe, fresh fruit; the sensual kneading and shaping of bread dough; the careful placement of mounds of cookie batter on well-greased baking sheets; and the pleasure in decorating a pie or cake to delight those who would taste it first with their eyes.

Of course, like so many other women, I didn't always have time during my early years as a wife and mother to devote time to baking as my mother had done. For special occasions, of course, I would open up my box of handwritten recipes and prove I was truly my mother's daughter when it came to baking from scratch!

But as the children grew older and I became a single parent, I found myself baking less and less. I was working full-time and going to college, and it was easier just to pick up sweets from the store or a bakery. What started as a convenience became a tough habit to break, and eating all those sugar-filled, high-fat goodies ultimately began to put my health at risk.

Baking the Healthy Exchanges Way

I figured I could give up all things sweet for a little while—while I was on a *diet*. But to lose weight once and for all, and to keep it off for a lifetime, I needed to find new ways to eat and new ways to bake. I had to reinvent the recipes I loved so I could continue eating the foods I loved without compromising my health.

That's how Healthy Exchanges was born all those years ago, and that has been at the heart of everything I've done since then. Baking the Healthy Exchanges Way has essentially let me "have my cake and eat it, too." It's allowed me to remain connected to my beloved family traditions *without* having to live with food-related medical concerns.

That's not to say it was easy baking in this new way. One of the greatest challenges I faced when I began was figuring out what sweetener to use—and how to cope with the ways it baked up differently than traditional sugar. The same was true with the various low-fat and fat-free shortening choices. Each recipe I created and baked with these ever-changing new products taught me something else. Over the years, I've learned a lot about what works—and what doesn't. Now I'm passing all that precious knowledge along to you.

> "Families are like fudge . . . mostly sweet with a few nuts."
> —Author unknown

Nothing but the Best

Now, one of the most important things I've learned about baking along the way is never to skimp on equipment. That means I'm giving you permission to empty your kitchen cabinets of bent and warped cookie sheets, blackened baking pans, springform pans that have lost their shape, and pie plates that have become so discolored from use that no amount of scrubbing can return them to their original glory.

I'm not just talking about pans, either. I want you to act like an archeologist and go deep into your utensil drawer or bin. Is the rubber on your spatula worn and rubbed down? Toss it into the nearest wastebasket! Is your only whisk a scrawny, cheap one that doesn't have the strength to handle cream cheese for cheesecakes? You deserve something better! Treat yourself to a big, beautiful mixing bowl—the largest one that will fit in your cabinet, if possible! And if you're still using the old 2-cup glass measuring cup you got from your grandmother or a yard sale ten years ago, I want you to consider upgrading your baking tools. Invest in good measuring cups (with the quantities clearly written so that it's easy to see how much you have) for both liquid and dry ingredients. Good measuring cups are *never* a luxury. (I like having extra sets of the dry cups, so if I have to measure one cup of two items in a recipe, I don't have to wash the cup out and dry it completely before using it again.)

It makes a difference, it really does. For one thing, you're simply able to do the necessary jobs more skillfully, whether it's measuring ingredients accurately, stirring the right amount of air into a dough (but not too much), or scraping every last bit of batter from your bowl into your baking pan with a spatula that has a clean, sharp edge to it—and no musty, rubbery smell!

And, speaking of bowls: People used to tease me when I traveled to cooking demos with my own 8-cup Pyrex measuring cup/mixing bowl (and my own whisk) in my carry-on bag, but I learned the hard way not to take a chance that I wouldn't have what I needed to prepare my recipe in front of an audience. When you've learned what works for you, always use it. Your confidence will grow by leaps and bounds—and you'll know that you'll get a good result every time!

I've shared tips on equipment in each of the following chapters, so make certain you read those sections completely before stirring up any of the recipes. But understand that your results may still vary. Every oven is different, and even variables like humidity, altitude, and time of day can make a difference in your dish. Don't worry about it, but pay close attention to how a recipe bakes up. If something browns too quickly, your oven may be hotter than the knobs indicate. You can check this with an oven thermometer, but in the meantime, adjust the temperature and/or the cooking time as needed.

Do you live at sea level or up in the mountains? That also can make a difference in how your recipe turns out. If your home is in Denver, the Mile High City, you may have already learned that your thinner air can make cakes rise too quickly or your liquids evaporate too much, producing a flatter or drier result. One website I consulted recently noted that pioneer cooks used to solve altitude problems by adding an egg to a recipe designed to be baked at sea level. Interesting, right? And maybe worth some experimenting, if you've experienced problems like this.

I'm often asked about new kinds of baking equipment (like some of the new flexible silicone bakeware), and while I'm as curious as the next cook and have tried some of them out myself, I still base my carefully tested recipes on standard metal cooking pans. So don't feel you've got to run out and buy all new pans, as long as the ones you have are in good condition. But if you've got a birthday coming up and you love the idea of a muffin pan that nothing sticks to, put one on your wish list!

"If you have a burning, restless urge to write or paint, simply eat something sweet and the feeling will pass."
—Fran Lebowitz

Baking Is Creative

Another reason I believe that baking is back in America is the growing trend toward creative pastimes, maybe as a counterpoint to our increased interest in and dependence on technology. Everywhere you look, people are knitting, scrapbooking, giving their homes an "extreme makeover"—and reveling in the creative outlets these pursuits offer.

Baking fits in perfectly with the rest of these activities because it's *personal*. You choose the recipe, adjust it to your own or your family's particular likes and dislikes, select the menu that will incorporate it, and then prepare it with your own hands. Even when you use handy, healthy convenience foods to decrease your actual time in the kitchen, you're still creating something special—something that says "I care about you" to the people who share your table.

Baking is also a wonderful activity to do together—parents with children, grandparents with grandkids, and even older children with younger ones. It's a great opportunity to pass along family history while preparing a recipe that's been handed down from generation to generation; it's also a chance to help young children learn measurement math and plenty of new vocabulary words! There's so much learning that goes on in the kitchen, and because it occurs in an informal setting, the chefs (young and old) are relaxed and open to deepening their relationships with one another.

Baking in Grandma JO's Kitchen

I know that many people aren't fortunate enough to have a grandmother to teach them how to bake; many others don't have an old wooden recipe box (or a tin one, like Barbara's mom) filled with dog-eared, fading, grease-stained recipe cards that tell the long and irresistible story of a family and food. That's where I come in!

I've come to consider myself *everyone's* grandma, and I'm inviting you to join me in my comfortable and cozy farm kitchen. You can be sure that I'll always share the best of my stories and secrets, my techniques and tips. With my help you can enjoy fresh and tasty baked goods at your house—and be reassured that all that homemade goodness also happens to be good for you!

When I was younger, I don't think I thought very much about my legacy, what I'd leave behind someday when I relocated to Cookbook Heaven, but in recent years, I've realized that I care very much about passing along the kitchen wisdom of my mother and grandmothers, as well as my own. I've been blessed to share what I know with my own wonderful children and grandchildren, but my kitchen—and my heart—is big enough to make room for you and your family, too!

Jo Anna

"That it will never come again
Is what makes life so sweet."
—Emily Dickinson

Please note:

In many of my cookbooks, I've included my Healthy Exchanges eating plan, which explains how to use my version of the "exchange" system for planning what to eat and how much to eat for optimum health and weight loss (or maintenance). Because this is a "special-interest" cookbook, I've chosen to focus just on the recipes in this volume. If this is your first Healthy Exchanges cookbook, please check one of my other books for an explanation of the exchange system and an abundance of healthy cooking tips! Good recent choices include *The Open Road Cookbook* or *Cooking Healthy with a Man in Mind.*

A Peek into
My *Baking with*
Splenda Pantry

In most of my books, I've included a comprehensive list of brands I've tested and prefer in just about every aisle of the supermarket. But for this special book, I decided to share *only* the products that I used for these recipes. I wanted you to be able to get the same great results I did when you prepare these dishes. If you're unable to find one of these products or you prefer another to my choice, please understand that you may not achieve the same results that I did.

Fat-free plain yogurt (*Dannon*)
Nonfat dry milk powder (*Carnation*)
Evaporated fat-free milk (*Carnation*)
No-fat sour cream (*Land O Lakes*)
Fat-free half & half (*Land O Lakes*)
Fat-free cream cheese (*Philadelphia*)
Reduced-calorie margarine (*I Can't Believe It's Not Butter! Light*)
Reduced-calorie whipped topping (*Cool Whip Lite or Cool Whip Free*)
Biscuit baking mix (*Bisquick Reduced Fat*)
All-purpose flour (*Pillsbury*)
Cake flour (*Swan's Down*)
Bread machine flour (*Pillsbury*)

Dry yeast (*Red Star or Fleischmann's*)
Purchased piecrust
  Unbaked (*Pillsbury—in the dairy case*)
  Graham-cracker, shortbread and chocolate (*Keebler*)
Quick oats (*Quaker Oats*)
Graham-cracker crumbs (*Nabisco Honey Maid*)
Baking powder (*Calumet*)
Baking soda (*Arm & Hammer*)
Cornstarch (*Argo*)
Unsweetened cocoa powder (*Hershey's Cocoa*)
Unsweetened chocolate squares (*Baker's*)
Mini chocolate chips (*Hershey's*)
Reduced-calorie chocolate syrup (*Hershey's Lite Syrup*)
Sugar-free pancake syrup (*Log Cabin*)
Reduced-fat peanut butter (*Peter Pan, Jif, or Skippy*)
Pie filling (*Lucky Leaf No Sugar Added Cherry and Apple*)
Unsweetened applesauce (*Musselman's*)
Unsweetened apple juice (*Musselman's*)
Unsweetened orange juice (*Simply Orange*)
Reduced-calorie cranberry juice cocktail (*Ocean Spray*)
Lemon and lime juice (*ReaLemon or ReaLime—in plastic lemon
  and lime containers*)
Raisins and mixed fruit bits (*Sun-Maid*)
Craisins (*Ocean Spray*)
Dried apricots (*Sunsweet*)
Flaked coconut (*Baker's Angel Flake*)
Sugar-free gelatin and puddings (*JELL-O*)
Sugar-free and fat-free ice cream (*Wells' Blue Bunny*)
Spreadable fruit spread (*Welch's or Smucker's*)
Wafer cookies (*Murry's Sugar Free*)
Sugar-free peppermint candies (*Bob's Sugar Free Starlight
  Mints*)
Diet lemon-lime soda pop (*Diet Mountain Dew*)
Diet white grape soda pop (*Diet Rite*)
Cooking spray (*Pam butter-flavored or Pam for Baking with
  Flour*)

JoAnna's Ten Commandments of Successful Cooking

A very important part of any journey is knowing where you are going and the best way to get there. If you plan and prepare before you start to cook, you should reach mealtime with foods to write home about!

1. **Read the entire recipe from start to finish** and be sure you understand the process involved. Check that you have all the equipment you will need *before* you begin.

2. **Check the ingredients list** and be sure you have *everything*, and in the amounts required. Keep cooking sprays handy—while they're not listed as ingredients, I use them all the time (just a quick squirt!).

3. **Set out *all* the ingredients and equipment needed** to prepare the recipe on the counter near you *before* you start. Remember that old saying, *A stitch in time saves nine?* It applies in the kitchen, too.

4. **Do as much advance preparation as possible** before actually cooking. Chop, cut, grate, or do whatever is

needed to prepare the ingredients and have them ready before you start to mix. Turn the oven on at least ten minutes before putting food in to bake, to allow the oven to preheat to the proper temperature.

5. **Use a kitchen timer** to tell you when the cooking or baking time is up. Because stove temperatures vary slightly by manufacturer, you may want to set your timer for five minutes less than the suggested time to prevent overcooking. Check the progress of your dish at that time, then decide whether or not you need the additional minutes.

6. **Measure carefully.** Use glass measures for liquids, and metal or plastic cups for dry ingredients. My recipes are based on standard measurements. Unless I tell you it's a scant or full cup, measure the cup level.

7. **For best results, follow the recipe instructions exactly.** Feel free to substitute ingredients that *don't tamper* with the basic chemistry of the recipe, but be sure to leave key ingredients alone. For example, you could substitute sugar-free instant chocolate pudding for sugar-free instant butterscotch pudding, but if you use a six-serving package when a four-serving package was listed in the ingredients, or if you use instant when cook-and-serve is required, you won't get the right result.

8. **Clean up as you go.** It is much easier to wash a few items at a time than to face a whole counter of dirty dishes later. The same is true for spills on the counter or floor.

9. **Be careful about doubling or halving a recipe.** Though many recipes can be altered successfully to serve more or fewer people, *many cannot.* This is especially true when it comes to spices and liquids. If you try to double a recipe that calls for 1 teaspoon pumpkin-pie spice, for example, and you double the spice, you may end up with a too-spicy taste. I usually suggest increasing spices or liquid by 1½ times when doubling a recipe. If it tastes a little bland to you, you can increase the spice to 1¾ times the origi-

nal amount the next time you prepare the dish. Remember: You can always add more, but you can't take it out after it's stirred in.

The same is true with liquid ingredients. If you wanted to *triple* a main dish recipe because you were planning to serve a crowd, you might think you should use three times as much of every ingredient. Don't, or you could end up with soup instead! If the original recipe calls for 1¾ cup tomato sauce, I'd suggest using 3½ cups when you **triple** the recipe (or 2¾ cups if you **double** it). You'll still have a good-tasting dish that won't run all over the plate.

10. **Write your reactions next to each recipe once you've served it.** Yes, that's right, I'm giving you permission to write in this book. It's yours, after all. Ask yourself: Did everyone like it? Did you have to add another half teaspoon of chili seasoning to please your family, who like to live on the spicier side of the street? You may even want to rate the recipe on a scale of 1☆ to 4☆, depending on what you thought of it. (Four stars would be the top rating—and I hope you'll feel that way about many of my recipes.) Jotting down your comments while they are fresh in your mind will help you personalize the recipe to your own taste the next time you prepare it.

The Recipes

How to Read a Healthy Exchanges Recipe

The Healthy Exchanges Nutritional Analysis

Before using these recipes, you may wish to consult your physician or health-care provider to be sure they are appropriate for you. The information in this book is not intended to take the place of any medical advice. It reflects my experiences, studies, research, and opinions regarding healthy eating.

Each recipe includes nutritional information calculated in three ways:

> Healthy Exchanges Weight Loss Choices™ or Exchanges
> Calories; Fat, Protein, Carbohydrates, and Fiber in grams;
>   Sodium and Calcium in milligrams
> Diabetic Exchanges

In every Healthy Exchanges recipe, the Diabetic Exchanges have been calculated by a registered dietitian. All the other calculations were done by computer, using the Food Processor II software.

When the ingredient listing gives more than one choice, the first ingredient listed is the one used in the recipe analysis. Due to inevitable variations in the ingredients you choose to use, the nutritional values should be considered approximate.

The annotation "(limited)" following Protein counts in some recipes indicates that consumption of whole eggs should be limited to four per week.

Please note the following symbols:

☆ This star means read the recipe's directions carefully for special instructions about **division** of ingredients.

❄ This symbol indicates FREEZES WELL.

And whenever you see a *HINT* that directs you to a Grandma JO recipe, please turn to the last chapter to find it.

Yummy Yeast

Breads

Did you know that yeast breads, made of dough that rises, go all the way back to ancient Egypt around 4000 BC? (The Internet is wonderful for digging up fascinating facts like that one!) In the years since then, bread has been an important part of the menu in almost every culture around the world. And because the manufacturers of bread machines have now made it incredibly easy to bake bread anytime at all, there's just no reason not to build a repertoire of breads you and your family love!

I'm ready to get you started on that little project, with this chapter of excellent yeast breads for every occasion. You can start with some beautiful basics like *Light Rye Bread* or *Basic Whole Wheat Bread*, then run a little wild with inventive delights like *Sour Cream Cornmeal Bread*, *Onion Dill Rye Bread*, and *Sweet Potato Bread*. As the saying goes, bread is the staff of life—and it's also at the heart of a healthy life!

Bread Machine Cooking Tips

I shared a number of cooking tips about baking in a bread machine in *JoAnna's Kitchen Miracles*, my book about seven truly marvelous kitchen machines that make cooking and baking the joy that it is today. What I learned on that book is still mostly true about the recipes in this book, but you'll see that Splenda changes things enough for me to alert you to the differences.

1. Not all bread machines are created equal! If you have an older model, you probably only have a 1-pound or 1½-pound setting. The newer models with all their bells and whistles have settings for 1-pound, 1½-pound, and even 2-pound loaves! I've decided to concentrate on the 1½-pound loaf in my recipes, because this is the loaf size most folks are interested in baking. As my Diabetic Exchanges have to come out right in addition to the bread, this size loaf seems to be perfect for both those needs. (Speaking of older and new models: If you're thinking of replacing your current machine or you're in the market for the first time, I suggest getting a machine that bakes the bread horizontally instead of vertically. Our recipe testing demonstrated that "longer" is better than "taller" for baking bread this way.)

2. Be sure to read your bread machine's manual from start to finish at least once before using any of my recipes, so you are familiar with the "add ingredients" feature and everything else about your machine. This is the first step in ensuring bread-baking success!

3. This advice is so important, I'm going to repeat it: Read your bread machine's manual from start to finish before using any of my recipes.

4. Since homemade bread does not contain preservatives, loaves will usually stay fresh for only a couple of days. If you know that you'll not be using it all up in that time, why don't you cut the loaf into the suggested 12 slices after it's cooled and freeze the slices in individual plastic zipper bags? Two slices to a bag is a nice number. Freeze for up to two months. When thawing, place the freezer bag on a plate and let set for 2 hours OR open the top of the bag, place the bag on a paper plate and microwave on HIGH for about 15 to 20 seconds.

5. Recently, bread-machine yeast has found its way to the marketplace. When first starting to test these recipes, I chose to test the bread baked both with bread-machine

yeast and with regular dry yeast. We did NOT find a noticeable difference in either taste or texture in my bread recipes using either, so this is a personal choice left up to you. Often, the bread-machine yeast costs a bit more than the dry bottled yeast. However, the most expensive of all yeast are the little individual paper packets, which contain ¼ ounce (2¼ teaspoons) of dry yeast. My choice is to buy my yeast in jars.

6. In all my bread-machine recipes, I call for bread flour, which is great for bread machines. Why, you ask? Because bread flour is made from hard spring wheat and contains a higher percentage of protein than regular all-purpose flour, and helps give the finished loaf a more even texture. At least half the flour in my recipe is bread flour—with the remainder usually being whole-wheat or rye. This combination helps to ensure success with your finished product.

7. Make sure both your yeast and your flour stay fresh. I often buy in bulk and then store both the yeast and the flour in my freezer. I place each in a Zip-loc freezer bag and store them in the same general area of my freezer. Then, whenever I want to make a loaf of bread, I know that I won't have to drive into town to get my yeast and flour. All I have to do is go to my freezer! After deciding to make a loaf of bread, I take my flour and yeast from the freezer, get my bread machine out of the cupboard, and gather together all the remaining ingredients needed for the recipe. By the time I'm ready to put the flour and yeast into the machine, both have warmed to room temperature and work beautifully. A good, quality bread-machine flour will keep for up to two years in the freezer, and the yeast for at least one year.

8. Speaking of room temperature—bread recipes turn out best when all the ingredients are at room temperature, especially the liquids. If, after gathering everything together, the liquids are still too cold, I put them in a

small container and warm them up in my microwave for 30 to 60 seconds on HIGH. You don't want them hot—just warmed to that proverbial "room temperature"! The only exceptions to this are ingredients that are normally stored in the refrigerator, such as milk, sour cream, and eggs.

9. I've found that the best way to measure flour is to stir it with a spoon first. This aerates the flour and makes for more accurate measuring. Lightly spoon the aerated flour into your measuring cup. Do not tap the sides of the cup to pack it down. Level the flour with a butter knife or spatula. I know this seems like a bit of fuss for one of my recipes, but this technique ensures that you don't use too much flour, and, therefore, you won't be baking yeast bricks instead of bread.

10. Salt is an essential part of the bread-making process. The amount needed is so small that it really doesn't amount to a "hill of salt" in the end. Don't skip this vital ingredient or your bread will not turn out correctly.

11. It's very important to measure all ingredients correctly BEFORE adding them to the machine. It's a case of doing like the carpenter—measure with your eyes twice, pour once. Sometimes, adding as little as one tablespoon too much liquid can make the difference between a perfect loaf of bread and an "also ran" loaf.

12. Heavy-texture breads, such as whole wheat, do not rise as high as a basic white bread, especially if fruits or nuts or such are part of the recipe.

13. Hot, humid weather or extra-cold, windy days can affect the outcome of your bread, so try not to do the prep work near a window. Early morning works best for those sticky summer days. Later in the day, when the temperature is usually warmer, is better for winter months. It may sound silly to check the weather before turning on your machine, but you'll thank me when your bread turns out properly.

14. As the number of bread machines and the differences in homes and temperature conditions are as varied as the stars in heaven, I suggest that the first time you try a new bread-machine recipe, you watch and listen carefully to your machine. Check the dough after the first 3 to 5 minutes. If your machine sounds like it's working too hard during the mixing cycle *or* if the dough looks dry and crumbly *or* if two or more balls of dough form, then add additional liquid (water) a teaspoon at a time until one smooth ball forms. If the dough has too much moisture and does not form a ball, add additional bread flour a tablespoon at a time until a smooth ball forms. Be sure to keep a record of this on the recipe page. Bread dough with the correct amount of flour and liquid for the conditions of the machine will form a smooth ball before starting the baking cycle.

15. But—open the lid of the bread machine ONLY during the mixing and kneading stages. If you open the machine during the rising or baking cycles, the loaf will almost always collapse.

"Homemade" White Bread

Want the taste of delectable homemade bread with all the ease of today's modern kitchen magicians? Here's my version, made especially good with just a touch of Splenda.   ☻   Serves 12

> ¾ cup water
> 6 tablespoons fat-free half & half
> 2 tablespoons reduced-calorie margarine
> 3 cups bread flour
> 2 tablespoons SPLENDA Granular
> 1½ teaspoons table salt
> 1 tablespoon active dry yeast

In a bread-machine container, combine water, half & half, and margarine. Add bread flour, Splenda, and salt. Make an indentation on top of dry ingredients. Pour yeast into indentation. Follow your bread machine's instructions for a 1½-pound loaf. Remove loaf from machine and place on a wire rack to cool. Cut into 12 slices. Makes one (1½-pound) loaf.

Each serving equals:

HE: 1½ Bread • ¼ Fat • 5 Optional Calories

133 Calories • 1 gm Fat • 5 gm Protein • 26 gm Carbohydrate • 302 mg Sodium • 13 mg Calcium • 1 gm Fiber

DIABETIC EXCHANGES: 1½ Starch

Egg Bread

Does it surprise you to find a recipe for bread containing eggs? You'll find that they produce a gorgeously golden loaf that tastes remarkably rich! This bread is also great for making French toast.

Serves 12

> 2 eggs, or equivalent in egg substitute
> ¾ cup fat-free half & half
> 1 tablespoon + 1 teaspoon reduced-calorie margarine
> 3 cups bread flour
> 3 tablespoons SPLENDA Granular
> 1½ teaspoons table salt
> 2 teaspoons active dry yeast

In a bread-machine container, combine eggs, half & half, and margarine. Add bread flour, Splenda, and salt. Make an indentation on top of dry ingredients. Pour yeast into indentation. Follow your bread machine's instructions for a 1½-pound loaf. Remove loaf from machine and place on a wire rack to cool. Cut into 12 slices. Makes one (1½-pound) loaf.

Each serving equals:

HE: 1½ **Bread** • ¼ **Slider** • 6 **Optional Calories**

146 Calories • 2 gm Fat • 6 gm Protein • 26 gm Carbohydrate • 332 mg Sodium • 25 mg Calcium • 1 gm Fiber

DIABETIC EXCHANGES: 1½ **Starch**

Basic Whole Wheat Bread

Every baker should have a few reliable recipe classics in her repertoire, and this is one of my favorite "basics"! Make sure your flour hasn't been sitting for months in your kitchen cabinets—fresh tastes best.   ☺   Serves 12

> ¾ cup water
> 6 tablespoons fat-free milk
> 2 tablespoons reduced-calorie margarine
> 1 cup whole wheat flour
> 2 cups bread flour
> 2 tablespoons SPLENDA Granular
> 1½ teaspoons table salt
> 2¼ teaspoons active dry yeast

In a bread-machine container, combine water, milk, and margarine. Add whole wheat flour, bread flour, Splenda, and salt. Make an indentation on top of dry ingredients. Pour yeast into indentation. Follow your bread machine's instructions for a 1½-pound loaf. Remove loaf from machine and place on a wire rack to cool. Cut into 12 slices. Makes one (1½-pound) loaf.

Each serving equals:

HE: 1½ Bread • ¼ Fat • 3 Optional Calories

125 Calories • 1 gm Fat • 4 gm Protein • 25 gm Carbohydrate • 295 mg Sodium • 17 mg Calcium • 2 gm Fiber

DIABETIC EXCHANGES: 1½ Starch

Maple Wheat Bread

If you love the taste of maple syrup (and who doesn't?) but don't serve pancakes often enough to please your taste buds, try stirring a little "New England gold" into a loaf of wheat bread. Scrumptious!

❍ Serves 12

   ⅓ cup fat-free milk
   ⅔ cup sugar-free maple syrup
   ¼ cup water
   2 tablespoons reduced-calorie margarine
   1 cup whole wheat flour
   2 cups bread flour
   2 tablespoons SPLENDA Granular
   1 teaspoon table salt
   1 tablespoon active dry yeast

In a bread-machine container, combine milk, maple syrup, water, and margarine. Add whole wheat flour, bread flour, Splenda, and salt. Make an indentation on top of dry ingredients. Pour yeast into indentation. Follow your bread machine's instructions for a 1½-pound loaf. Remove loaf from machine and place on a wire rack to cool. Cut into 12 slices. Makes one (1½-pound) loaf.

Each serving equals:

HE: 1½ Bread • ¼ Fat • 11 Optional Calories

137 Calories • 1 gm Fat • 5 gm Protein • 27 gm Carbohydrate • 243 mg Sodium • 16 mg Calcium • 2 gm Fiber

DIABETIC EXCHANGES: 1½ Starch

Whole Wheat Molasses Bread

Molasses has such a strong flavor, you need only a touch of it to transform a plain loaf of wheat bread into hearty country fare. It tastes so good, it's almost like cake! ☻ Serves 12

1 cup + 1 tablespoon water
1 tablespoon vegetable oil
2 tablespoons molasses
2 cups bread flour
1 cup whole wheat flour
2 tablespoons SPLENDA Granular
1 teaspoon table salt
2¼ teaspoons active dry yeast

In a bread-machine container, combine water, vegetable oil, and molasses. Add bread flour, whole wheat flour, Splenda, and salt. Make an indentation on top of dry ingredients. Pour yeast into indentation. Follow your bread machine's instructions for a 1½-pound loaf. Remove loaf from machine and place on a wire rack to cool. Cut into 12 slices. Makes one (1½-pound) loaf.

Each serving equals:

HE: 1½ Bread • ¼ Fat • 11 Optional Calories

142 Calories • 2 gm Fat • 4 gm Protein • 27 gm Carbohydrate • 196 mg Sodium • 14 mg Calcium • 2 gm Fiber

DIABETIC EXCHANGES: 1½ Starch

Walnut Whole Wheat Bread

Why put the cream cheese *in* the bread instead of on top? Good question. Blending cream cheese into the dough makes it incredibly luscious, and the walnuts provide a terrific touch of crunch.

○ Serves 12

> 1 (8-ounce) package fat-free cream cheese
> ¾ cup water
> 1 tablespoon + 1 teaspoon reduced-calorie margarine
> 1 cup whole wheat flour
> 2 cups bread flour
> 3 tablespoons SPLENDA Granular
> 1½ teaspoons table salt
> 2¼ teaspoons active dry yeast
> ½ cup chopped walnuts

In a bread-machine container, stir cream cheese with a sturdy spoon until soft. Stir in water and margarine. Add whole-wheat flour, bread flour, Splenda, and salt. Make an indentation on top of ingredients. Pour yeast into indentation. Follow your bread machine's instructions for a 1½-pound loaf. Add walnuts when "add ingredient" signal beeps. Continue following your machine's instructions until the bread is finished. Remove loaf from machine and place on a wire rack to cool. Cut into 12 slices. Makes one (1½-pound) loaf.

Each serving equals:

HE: 1½ Bread • ½ Protein • ½ Fat • 2 Optional Calories

159 Calories • 3 gm Fat • 7 gm Protein • 26 gm Carbohydrate • 410 mg Sodium • 45 mg Calcium • 2 gm Fiber

DIABETIC EXCHANGES: 1½ Starch • 1 Fat

Light Rye Bread

Light in color, light in flavor, and a de-light that originated in Eastern Europe, this rye bread makes wonderful sandwiches. If you don't care for caraway seeds, it's possible to make this bread without them—but they add so much intense flavor, I recommend you give them a try. ☻ Serves 12

> 1 cup + 2 tablespoons flat, light, nonalcoholic beer
> 2 tablespoons vegetable oil
> ¾ cup rye flour
> 2¼ cups bread flour
> 2 tablespoons SPLENDA Granular
> 1½ teaspoons caraway seeds
> 1½ teaspoons table salt
> 2¼ teaspoons active dry yeast

In a bread-machine container, combine beer and vegetable oil. Add rye flour, bread flour, Splenda, caraway seeds, and salt. Make an indentation on top of dry ingredients. Pour yeast into indentation. Follow your bread machine's instructions for a 1½-pound loaf. Remove loaf from machine and place on a wire rack to cool. Cut into 12 slices. Makes one (1½-pound) loaf.

Each serving equals:

HE: 1½ Bread • ½ Fat • 5 Optional Calories

143 Calories • 3 gm Fat • 4 gm Protein • 25 gm Carbohydrate • 292 mg Sodium • 8 mg Calcium • 2 gm Fiber

DIABETIC EXCHANGES: 1½ Starch • ½ Fat

Swedish Rye Bread

Don't let this list of ingredients discourage you from putting this tangy bread on the menu soon. The end result is SO worth it! It's not only nutritious (with carrots, orange juice), but delicious, too.

◖ Serves 12

> ½ cup fat-free half & half
> ⅓ cup water
> 1 tablespoon unsweetened orange juice
> 2 tablespoons vegetable oil
> 2 tablespoons molasses
> 1 cup rye flour
> 2 cups bread flour
> 2 tablespoons SPLENDA Granular
> ⅓ cup grated carrots
> ½ teaspoon ground nutmeg
> 1½ teaspoons table salt
> 2¼ teaspoons active dry yeast

In a bread-machine container, combine half & half, water, orange juice, vegetable oil, and molasses. Add rye flour, bread flour, Splenda, carrots, nutmeg, and salt. Make an indentation on top of dry ingredients. Pour yeast into indentation. Follow your bread machine's instructions for a 1½-pound loaf. Remove loaf from machine and place on a wire rack to cool. Cut into 12 slices. Makes one (1½-pound) loaf.

Each serving equals:

HE: 1½ Bread • ½ Fat • 18 Optional Calories

138 Calories • 2 gm Fat • 4 gm Protein • 26 gm Carbohydrate • 309 mg Sodium • 20 mg Calcium • 2 gm Fiber

DIABETIC EXCHANGES: 1½ Starch • ½ Fat

Cliff's Rye Bread

My husband, Cliff, the truck drivin' man, has eaten his way across this nation, and he's tasted outstanding breads from every state and region. When I was creating recipes for this chapter, I decided to invent one inspired by the flavorful rye bread he's enjoyed on the East Coast. ○ Serves 12

⅓ cup fat-free milk
¾ cup water
2 tablespoons reduced-calorie margarine
1 cup rye flour
2 cups bread flour
2 tablespoons SPLENDA Granular
1½ teaspoons table salt
1 tablespoon active dry yeast

In a bread-machine container, combine milk, water, and margarine. Add rye flour, bread flour, Splenda, and salt. Make an indentation on top of dry ingredients. Pour yeast into indentation. Follow your bread machine's instructions for a 1½-pound loaf. Remove loaf from machine and place on a wire rack to cool. Cut into 12 slices. Makes one (1½-pound) loaf.

Each serving equals:

HE: 1½ Bread • ¼ Fat • 3 Optional Calories

121 Calories • 1 gm Fat • 4 gm Protein • 24 gm Carbohydrate • 317 mg Sodium • 15 mg Calcium • 2 gm Fiber

DIABETIC EXCHANGES: 1½ Starch

"Buttermilk" Rye Bread

Classic rye bread has a bit of a "sour" taste, so buttermilk is a perfect ingredient to help achieve that flavor. It's acidic instead of buttery, but it makes truly appetizing bread. ❂ Serves 12

> 1 cup nonfat dry milk powder
> 1 cup + 2 tablespoons water
> 1 tablespoon white distilled vinegar
> 2 tablespoons vegetable oil
> 2 tablespoons molasses
> 2 cups bread flour
> 1 cup rye flour
> 2 tablespoons SPLENDA Granular
> 2 teaspoons caraway seeds
> ¼ teaspoon baking soda
> 1½ teaspoons table salt
> 2½ teaspoons active dry yeast

In a bread-machine container, combine dry milk powder, water, and vinegar. Let set for 5 minutes. Stir in vegetable oil and molasses. Add bread flour, rye flour, Splenda, caraway seeds, baking soda, and salt. Make an indentation on top of dry ingredients. Pour yeast into indentation. Follow your bread machine's instructions for a 1½-pound loaf. Remove loaf from machine and place on a wire rack to cool. Cut into 12 slices. Makes one (1½-pound) loaf.

Each serving equals:

HE: 1½ Bread • ½ Fat • ¼ Fat-Free Milk • 11 Optional Calories

167 Calories • 3 gm Fat • 6 gm Protein • 29 gm Carbohydrate • 350 mg Sodium • 91 mg Calcium • 2 gm Fiber

DIABETIC EXCHANGES: 1½ Starch • ½ Fat

Oatmeal Walnut Bread

On those mornings when you're rushing out the door and don't have time for a bowl of good-for-you oatmeal, why not grab a slice or two of this cozy bread? You'll be getting some milk, some oats, and some crunch from wonderful walnuts! ☾ Serves 12

¾ cup fat-free milk
⅓ cup water
2 tablespoons reduced-calorie margarine
2¼ cups bread flour
¾ cup quick oats
¼ cup SPLENDA Granular
1½ teaspoons table salt
2¼ teaspoons active dry yeast
½ cup chopped walnuts

In a bread-machine container, combine milk, water, and margarine. Add bread flour, oats, Splenda, and salt. Make an indentation on top of dry ingredients. Pour yeast into indentation. Follow your bread machine instructions for a 1½-pound loaf. Add walnuts when "add ingredient" signal beeps. Continue following your machine's instructions. Remove loaf from machine and place on a wire rack to cool. Cut into 12 slices. Makes one (1½-pound) loaf.

Each serving equals:

HE: 1½ Bread • ½ Fat • 15 Optional Calories

161 Calories • 5 gm Fat • 5 gm Protein • 24 gm Carbohydrate • 321 mg Sodium • 31 mg Calcium • 2 gm Fiber

DIABETIC EXCHANGES: 1½ Starch • ½ Fat

Almond-Poppy Seed Bread

For a change of pace, here's a bread with an unusual flavor and texture that may remind you of the exotic Middle East, where almonds and poppy seeds are staples. It has splendid texture, too, making it perfect to serve at brunch for friends.   ☻   Serves 12

1 egg, or equivalent in egg substitute
¾ cup fat-free milk
2 tablespoons reduced-calorie margarine
1½ teaspoons almond extract
2¼ cups bread flour
½ cup quick oats
¼ cup SPLENDA Granular
2 tablespoons poppy seeds
¾ teaspoon table salt
2¼ teaspoons active dry yeast
⅓ cup slivered almonds

In a bread-machine container, combine egg, milk, margarine, and almond extract. Add bread flour, oats, Splenda, poppy seeds, and salt. Make an indentation on top of dry ingredients. Pour yeast into indentation. Follow your bread machine's instructions for a 1½-pound loaf. Add almonds when "add ingredient" signal beeps. Continue following your machine's instructions. Remove loaf from machine and place on a wire rack to cool. Cut into 12 slices. Makes one (1½-pound) loaf.

Each serving equals:

HE: 1½ Bread • ½ Fat • ¼ Protein • 14 Optional Calories

144 Calories • 4 gm Fat • 6 gm Protein • 21 gm Carbohydrate • 181 mg Sodium •
53 mg Calcium • 2 gm Fiber

DIABETIC EXCHANGES: 1½ Starch • 1 Fat

Sweet Potato Bread

You can use canned or fresh-baked sweet potatoes in this recipe, but you may get a moister result with the canned variety. It produces a loaf of rich color and savory flavor; and it's great for serving alongside a hearty bowl of soup or stew.   ◐   Serves 12

> 1 cup cooked mashed sweet potatoes
> ½ cup + 1 tablespoon fat-free milk
> ¼ cup reduced-calorie margarine
> 3 cups bread flour
> ¼ cup SPLENDA Granular
> 1½ teaspoons table salt
> 1 tablespoon active dry yeast

In a bread-machine container, combine sweet potatoes, milk, and margarine. Add bread flour, Splenda, and salt. Make an indentation on top of dry ingredients. Pour yeast into indentation. Follow your bread machine's instructions for a 1½-pound loaf. Remove loaf from machine and place on a wire rack to cool. Cut into 12 slices. Makes one (1½-pound) loaf.

Each serving equals:

HE: 1½ Bread • ½ Fat • 5 Optional Calories

171 Calories • 3 gm Fat • 5 gm Protein • 31 gm Carbohydrate • 357 mg Sodium • 26 mg Calcium • 1 gm Fiber

DIABETIC EXCHANGES: 1½ Starch • ½ Fat

Sour Cream Cornmeal Bread

You might not expect sour cream and cornmeal to be perfect partners in bread baking, but each brings out the best in the other. Instead of dry and crumbly, this cornbread is lush and rich, ideal for serving with any Mexican-themed menu.   ☻   Serves 12

> ¾ cup fat-free sour cream
> ⅓ cup fat-free half & half
> 1 egg, or equivalent in egg substitute
> 2 tablespoons reduced-calorie margarine
> 2 tablespoons SPLENDA Granular
> 2¼ cups bread flour
> ¾ cup yellow cornmeal
> 1 teaspoon table salt
> 2 teaspoons active dry yeast

In a bread-machine container, combine sour cream, half & half, egg, and margarine. Add Splenda, bread flour, cornmeal, and salt. Make an indentation on top of dry ingredients. Pour yeast into indentation. Follow your bread machine's instructions for a 1½-pound loaf. Remove loaf from machine and place on a wire rack to cool. Cut into 12 slices. Makes one (1½-pound) loaf.

Each serving equals:

HE: 1½ Bread • ¼ Fat • 11 Optional Calories

154 Calories • 2 gm Fat • 5 gm Protein • 29 gm Carbohydrate • 253 mg Sodium • 34 mg Calcium • 1 gm Fiber

DIABETIC EXCHANGES: 1½ Starch

Oatmeal Sour Cream Bread

Here's another breakfast bread that will win applause when you serve it! Because it's made with oat bran and low-fat dairy products, it's a scrumptious choice for anyone concerned about cholesterol. But it doesn't taste dry and boring, as some "healthy" breads do.

● Serves 12

> ¾ cup fat-free sour cream
> ¼ cup fat-free milk
> ½ cup water
> 2 tablespoons reduced-calorie margarine
> ¾ cup quick oats
> ⅓ cup oat bran
> 2½ cups bread flour
> 3 tablespoons SPLENDA Granular
> 1 teaspoon baking soda
> 1½ teaspoons table salt
> 2¼ teaspoons active dry yeast

In a bread-machine container, combine sour cream, milk, water, and margarine. Add oats, oat bran, bread flour, Splenda, baking soda, and salt. Make an indentation on top of dry ingredients. Pour yeast into indentation. Follow your bread machine's instructions for a 1½-pound loaf. Remove loaf from machine and place on a wire rack to cool. Cut into 12 slices. Makes one (1½-pound) loaf.

Each serving equals:

HE: 1½ Bread • ¼ Fat • 18 Optional Calories

154 Calories • 2 gm Fat • 5 gm Protein • 29 gm Carbohydrate • 441 mg Sodium • 35 mg Calcium • 2 gm Fiber

DIABETIC EXCHANGES: 1½ Starch

Focaccia Bread

If you can't head to Italy tonight, I'll bring Italy to you instead! This bread delivers the unique herbs, spices, and cheese flavors of that irresistible Mediterranean country. Use good olive oil when you cook and bake, and you'll be much more satisfied with the dishes you prepare.　❂　Serves 12

1 cup water
2 tablespoons fat-free milk
3 tablespoons olive oil
3 cups bread flour
½ cup grated reduced-free Parmesan cheese
2 tablespoons SPLENDA Granular
2 teaspoons dried rosemary
1 teaspoon dried minced garlic
1 tablespoon dried onion flakes
1½ teaspoons table salt
2¼ teaspoons active dry yeast

In a bread-machine container, combine water, milk, and olive oil. Add bread flour, Parmesan cheese, Splenda, rosemary, garlic, onion flakes, and salt. Make an indentation on top of dry ingredients. Pour yeast into indentation. Follow your bread machine's instructions for a 1½-pound loaf. Remove loaf from machine and place on a wire rack to cool. Cut into 12 slices. Makes one (1½-pound) loaf.

Each serving equals:

HE: 1½ Bread • ¾ Fat • 19 Optional Calories

169 Calories • 5 gm Fat • 5 gm Protein • 26 gm Carbohydrate • 346 mg Sodium • 35 mg Calcium • 1 gm Fiber

DIABETIC EXCHANGES: 1½ Starch • 1 Fat

Pimiento Italian Bread

Long before your taste buds decide whether a dish is delicious, your eyes feast first—and that's why it's delightful to add a colorful element into a bread recipe! Here, those savory bits of red pimiento really raise spirits. ● Serves 12

> ¾ cup fat-free milk
> 2 tablespoons fat-free half & half
> 2 tablespoons water
> 3 tablespoons olive oil
> 3 cups bread flour
> 2 tablespoons SPLENDA Granular
> 1 teaspoon Italian seasoning
> 1 teaspoon table salt
> 2 teaspoons active dry yeast
> 2 (2-ounce) jars chopped pimiento, drained

In a bread-machine container, combine milk, half & half, water, and olive oil. Add bread flour, Splenda, Italian seasoning, and salt. Make an indentation on top of dry ingredients. Pour yeast into indentation. Follow your bread machine's instructions for a 1½-pound loaf. Add pimiento when "add ingredient" signal beeps. Continue following your machine's instructions. Remove loaf from machine and place on a wire rack to cool. Cut into 12 slices. Makes one (1½-pound) loaf.

Each serving equals:

HE: 1½ Bread • ¾ Fat • 8 Optional Calories

164 Calories • 4 gm Fat • 5 gm Protein • 27 gm Carbohydrate • 206 mg Sodium • 28 mg Calcium • 1 gm Fiber

DIABETIC EXCHANGES: 1½ Starch • 1 Fat

Herbed Cottage Cheese Bread

Fragrant as it bakes, and utterly delectable when it emerges from the bread machine, this appetizing loaf makes wonderful sandwiches and is especially good toasted! ❂ Serves 12

1 cup fat-free cottage cheese
1 egg, or equivalent in egg substitute
6 tablespoons water
2 tablespoons reduced-calorie margarine
3 cups bread flour
2 tablespoons SPLENDA Granular
½ teaspoon dried minced garlic
1 tablespoon Italian seasoning
1½ teaspoons table salt
2¼ teaspoons active dry yeast

In a bread-machine container, combine cottage cheese, egg, water, and margarine. Add bread flour, Splenda, garlic, Italian seasoning, and salt. Make an indentation on top of dry ingredients. Pour yeast into indentation. Follow your bread machine's instructions for a 1½-pound loaf. Remove loaf from machine and place on a wire rack to cool. Cut into 12 slices. Makes one (1½-pound) loaf.

Each serving equals:

HE: 1½ Bread • ¼ Protein • ¼ Fat • 1 Optional Calorie

129 Calories • 1 gm Fat • 7 gm Protein • 23 gm Carbohydrate • 393 mg Sodium • 17 mg Calcium • 1 gm Fiber

DIABETIC EXCHANGES: 1½ Starch

Zucchini Cottage Cheese Bread

We all need our vegetables, and this is a clever way to work some veggies into a yummy bread! Use your box grater for the zucchini if you like, though many cooks prefer to leave the work to a machine such as the Cuisinart. ☻ Serves 12

> 1 cup fat-free cottage cheese
> ¼ cup fat-free milk
> 2 tablespoons water
> 2 tablespoons reduced-calorie margarine
> ¾ cup grated raw zucchini
> 1 cup whole-wheat flour
> 2 cups bread flour
> 2 tablespoons SPLENDA Granular
> 1½ teaspoons table salt
> 2¼ teaspoons active dry yeast

In a bread-machine container, combine cottage cheese, milk, water, margarine, and zucchini. Add whole-wheat flour, bread flour, Splenda, and salt. Make an indentation on top of dry ingredients. Pour yeast into indentation. Follow your bread machine's instructions for a 1½-pound loaf. Remove loaf from machine and place on a wire rack to cool. Cut into 12 slices. Makes one (1½-pound) loaf.

Each serving equals:

HE: 1½ Bread • ¼ Fat • 16 Optional Calories

141 Calories • 1 gm Fat • 7 gm Protein • 26 gm Carbohydrate • 381 mg Sodium • 29 mg Calcium • 2 gm Fiber

DIABETIC EXCHANGES: 1½ Starch

Rosemary Sour Cream Whole Wheat Bread

This rich, savory bread is excellent for a dinner party or family gathering, good with or without a spread on top! This is a case when a dried herb is better for a recipe than fresh herbs from your window box would be. ☻ Serves 12

> ¾ cup fat-free sour cream
> 2 eggs, or equivalent in egg substitute
> 2 tablespoons water
> 2 tablespoons reduced-calorie margarine
> 1 cup whole wheat flour
> 2 cups bread flour
> 2 tablespoons SPLENDA Granular
> 2 teaspoons dried rosemary
> 1½ teaspoons table salt
> 2¼ teaspoons active dry yeast

In a bread-machine container, combine sour cream, eggs, water, and margarine. Add whole wheat flour, bread flour, Splenda, rosemary, and salt. Make an indentation on top of dry ingredients. Pour yeast into indentation. Follow your bread machine's instructions for a 1½-pound loaf. Remove loaf from machine and place on a wire rack to cool. Cut into 12 slices. Makes one (1½-pound) loaf.

Each serving equals:

HE: 1½ Bread • ¼ Fat • ¼ Slider • 8 Optional Calories

150 Calories • 2 gm Fat • 6 gm Protein • 27 gm Carbohydrate • 346 mg Sodium • 35 mg Calcium • 2 gm Fiber

DIABETIC EXCHANGES: 1½ Starch

Onion Dill Rye Bread

Not everyone is a fan of tangy bread, but this is a superb recipe to serve to your more adventurous friends and family members. If you've never baked with dill before, I think you'll be pleased at how much flavor it imparts. ❂   Serves 12

> 1 cup + 2 tablespoons water
> 3 tablespoons vegetable oil
> ¾ cup rye flour
> 2¼ cups bread flour
> 2 tablespoons SPLENDA Granular
> 1 tablespoon dried dill weed
> 2 tablespoons dried onion flakes
> 1½ teaspoons table salt
> 1 tablespoon active dry yeast

In a bread-machine container, combine water and vegetable oil. Add rye flour, bread flour, Splenda, dill weed, onion flakes, and salt. Make an indentation on top of dry ingredients. Pour yeast into indentation. Follow your bread machine's instructions for a 1½-pound loaf. Remove loaf from machine and place on a wire rack to cool. Cut into 12 slices. Makes one (1½-pound) loaf.

Each serving equals:

HE: 1½ Bread • ¾ Fat • 1 Optional Calorie

152 Calories • 4 gm Fat • 4 gm Protein • 25 gm Carbohydrate • 292 mg Sodium • 12 mg Calcium • 2 gm Fiber

DIABETIC EXCHANGES: 1½ Starch • ½ Fat

Apricot Graham Bread

I've often felt that apricots don't get the respect they deserve when it comes to baking. Dried, these luscious orange gems are available all year round, and they add lively sweetness to this comforting, fruity bread.　　❂　Serves 12

> 1 cup water
> 2 tablespoons vegetable oil
> 2 tablespoons molasses
> 2 cups bread flour
> ¾ cup whole wheat flour
> ¼ cup graham cracker crumbs
> 2 tablespoons SPLENDA Granular
> 3 tablespoons dry milk powder
> ¾ teaspoon table salt
> 2¼ teaspoons active dry yeast
> ½ cup coarsely chopped dried apricots

In a bread-machine container, combine water, vegetable oil, and molasses. Add bread flour, whole wheat flour, graham cracker crumbs, Splenda, dry milk powder, and salt. Make an indentation on top of dry ingredients. Pour yeast into indentation. Follow your bread machine's instructions for a 1½-pound loaf. Add apricots when "add ingredient" signal beeps. Continue following your machine's instructions. Remove loaf from machine and place on a wire rack to cool. Cut into 12 slices. Makes one (1½-pound) loaf.

Each serving equals:

HE: 1½ Bread • ½ Fat • ¼ Fruit • 15 Optional Calories

163 Calories • 3 gm Fat • 5 gm Protein • 29 gm Carbohydrate • 165 mg Sodium • 30 mg Calcium • 3 gm Fiber

DIABETIC EXCHANGES: 1½ Starch • ½ Fat

Apricot-Raisin Nut Bread

Dried fruit is a splendid secret when it comes to baking, because the heat and moisture of the baking process bring out all its intense, sweet flavor! This bread would make appealing tea sandwiches when spread with a flavored fat-free cream-cheese spread.

○ Serves 12

> 1 cup unsweetened apple juice
> 2 tablespoons reduced-calorie margarine
> 3 cups bread flour
> ⅓ cup SPLENDA Granular
> ½ teaspoon table salt
> 2¼ teaspoons active dry yeast
> ½ cup coarsely chopped dried apricots
> ½ cup seedless raisins
> 6 tablespoons coarsely chopped pecans

In a bread-machine container, combine apple juice and margarine. Add bread flour, Splenda, and salt. Make an indentation on top of dry ingredients. Pour yeast into indentation. Follow your bread machine's instructions for a 1½-pound loaf. Add apricots, raisins, and pecans when "add ingredient" signal beeps. Continue following your machine's instructions. Remove loaf from machine and place on a wire rack to cool. Cut into 12 slices. Makes one (1½-pound) loaf.

Each serving equals:

HE: 1½ Bread • ¾ Fruit • ¾ Fat • 2 Optional Calories

200 Calories • 4 gm Fat • 5 gm Protein • 36 gm Carbohydrate • 122 mg Sodium • 15 mg Calcium • 2 gm Fiber

DIABETIC EXCHANGES: 1½ Starch • 1 Fat • ½ Fruit

Zach's Cinnamon Raisin Bread

Raisin bread is one of the foods kids like best, and my grandson Zach is no exception! This bread was inspired by his love for raisins and cinnamon—a perfect pair, in his opinion.

○ Serves 12

> ¾ cup water
> ⅓ cup fat-free half & half
> 2 tablespoons + 2 teaspoons reduced-calorie margarine
> 2¼ cups bread flour
> ¾ cup whole-wheat flour
> ¼ cup SPLENDA Granular
> 2 teaspoons ground cinnamon
> ¾ teaspoon table salt
> 1 tablespoon active dry yeast
> ¾ cup seedless raisins

In a bread-machine container, combine water, half & half, and margarine. Add bread flour, whole-wheat flour, Splenda, cinnamon, and salt. Make an indentation on top of dry ingredients. Pour yeast into indentation. Follow your bread machine's instructions for a 1½-pound loaf. Add raisins when "add ingredient" signal beeps. Continue following your machine's instructions. Remove loaf from machine and place on a wire rack to cool. Cut into 12 slices. Makes one (1½-pound) loaf.

Each serving equals:

HE: 1½ Bread • ½ Fruit • ⅓ Fat • 6 Optional Calories

166 Calories • 2 gm Fat • 5 gm Protein • 32 gm Carbohydrate • 187 mg Sodium • 22 mg Calcium • 2 gm Fiber

DIABETIC EXCHANGES: 1½ Starch • ½ Fruit

Sunshine Bread

Give the day a great big culinary "good morning" when you serve this sunny bread, with tender raisins peeking out of each healthy slice! For a pretty change of pace, try golden raisins instead of the usual darker ones.   ● Serves 12

¾ cup fat-free sour cream
⅓ cup water
2 tablespoons reduced-calorie margarine
3 tablespoons dry oat bran hot cereal mix
¾ cup whole wheat flour
2¼ cups bread flour
¼ cup SPLENDA Granular
1 teaspoon table salt
2¼ teaspoons active dry yeast
½ cup seedless raisins
¼ cup sunflower seeds

In a bread-machine container, combine sour cream, water, and margarine. Add dry oat bran cereal mix, whole wheat flour, bread flour, Splenda, and salt. Make an indentation on top of dry ingredients. Pour yeast into indentation. Follow your bread machine's instructions for a 1½-pound loaf. Add raisins and sunflower seeds when "add ingredient" signal beeps. Continue following your machine's instructions. Remove loaf from machine and place on a wire rack to cool. Cut into 12 slices. Makes one (1½-pound) loaf.

Each serving equals:

HE: 1½ Bread • ½ Fat • ⅓ Fruit • ¼ Slider • 1 Optional Calorie

183 Calories • 3 gm Fat • 6 gm Protein • 33 gm Carbohydrate • 241 mg Sodium • 33 mg Calcium • 2 gm Fiber

DIABETIC EXCHANGES: 1½ Starch/Carbohydrate • 1½ Fat • ½ Fruit

Sour Cream–Raisin Spice Bread ❄

Here's a sweet and special bread that's a lovely choice for the holiday season but good all year long! Sour cream adds a luscious touch, and your kitchen will smell splendidly seductive as this bread bakes.   ☻   Serves 12

¾ cup fat-free sour cream
¾ cup water
2 tablespoons reduced-calorie margarine
3 cups bread flour
2 tablespoons SPLENDA Granular
1 tablespoon apple-pie spice
1½ teaspoons table salt
2 teaspoons active dry yeast
¾ cup seedless raisins

In a bread-machine container, combine sour cream, water, and margarine. Add bread flour, Splenda, apple-pie spice, and salt. Make an indentation on top of dry ingredients. Pour yeast into indentation. Follow your bread machine's instructions for a 1½-pound loaf. Add raisins when "add ingredient" signal beeps. Continue following your machine's instructions. Remove loaf from machine and place on a wire rack to cool. Cut into 12 slices. Makes one (1½-pound) loaf.

Each serving equals:

HE: 1½ Bread • ½ Fruit • ¼ Fat • 16 Optional Calories

174 Calories • 2 gm Fat • 5 gm Protein • 34 gm Carbohydrate • 335 mg Sodium • 33 mg Calcium • 1 gm Fiber

DIABETIC EXCHANGES: 1½ Starch • ½ Fruit

Coconut Banana Bran Bread

This taste-of-the-tropics recipe blends healthy oat bran cereal with a couple of nature's sweetest gifts—bananas and coconut! If a visit to Aruba isn't in your immediate future, you can close your eyes and imagine yourself breakfasting with this bread on a white sandy beach. ◑ Serves 12

> *1 egg, or equivalent in egg substitute*
> *½ cup fat-free half & half*
> *⅔ cup (2 medium) mashed ripe bananas*
> *2 tablespoons reduced-calorie margarine*
> *½ cup oat bran cereal*
> *¾ cup whole wheat flour*
> *2 cups bread flour*
> *¼ cup Splenda Granular*
> *1 teaspoon table salt*
> *2¼ teaspoons active dry yeast*
> *¼ cup flaked coconut*

In a bread-machine container, combine egg, half & half, bananas, and margarine. Add bran cereal, whole wheat flour, bread flour, Splenda, and salt. Make an indentation on top of dry ingredients. Pour yeast into indentation. Follow your bread machine's instructions for a 1½-pound loaf. Add coconut when "add ingredient" signal beefs. Continue following your machine's instructions. Remove loaf from machine and place on a wire rack to cool. Cut into 12 slices. Makes one (1½-pound) loaf.

Each serving equals:

HE: 1½ Bread • ⅓ Fruit • ¼ Fat • 19 Optional Calories

167 Calories • 3 gm Fat • 6 gm Protein • 29 gm Carbohydrate • 242 mg Sodium • 22 mg Calcium • 2 gm Fiber

DIABETIC EXCHANGES: 1½ Starch • ½ Fat

Cranberry Surprise Bread

Perhaps not all surprises are welcome, but this one definitely will be! As your family bites into a warm, inviting slice of this easy and scrumptious loaf, you're bound to see happy smiles all around.

○ Serves 12

1 cup unsweetened orange juice
2 tablespoons reduced-calorie margarine
3 cups bread flour
⅓ cup SPLENDA Granular
½ teaspoon ground nutmeg
¾ teaspoon table salt
2¼ teaspoons active dry yeast
½ cup chopped craisins
¼ cup chopped walnuts

In a bread-machine container, combine orange juice and margarine. Add flour, Splenda, nutmeg, and salt. Make an indentation on top of dry ingredients. Pour yeast into indentation. Follow your bread machine's instructions for a 1½-pound loaf. Add craisins and walnuts when "add ingredient" signal beeps. Continue following your machine's instructions. Remove loaf from machine and place on a wire rack to cool. Cut into 12 slices. Makes one (1½-pound) loaf.

Each serving equals:

HE: 1½ Bread • ½ Fruit • ⅓ Fat • 17 Optional Calories

175 Calories • 3 gm Fat • 5 gm Protein • 32 gm Carbohydrate • 169 mg Sodium • 10 mg Calcium • 2 gm Fiber

DIABETIC EXCHANGES: 1½ Starch • ½ Fruit • ½ Fat

Tropical Pineapple Bread

I've always believed in stirring in layers of flavors when I bake, and this bread illustrates that beautifully. The pineapple sends you winging toward those steamy, sultry islands—and the lemon-lime soda, coconut, and nuts bring you to a delicious happy landing!

○ Serves 12

> 1 (8-ounce) can crushed pineapple, packed in fruit juice, undrained
> ½ cup diet lemon-lime soda pop
> ⅓ cup fat-free half & half
> 2 tablespoons + 2 teaspoons reduced-calorie margarine
> ¾ cup whole wheat flour
> 2¼ cups bread flour
> ¼ cup SPLENDA Granular
> ½ teaspoon ground ginger
> ¼ teaspoon ground nutmeg
> 1 teaspoon table salt
> 2¼ teaspoons active dry yeast
> ¼ cup flaked coconut
> ¼ cup chopped macadamia nuts

In a bread-machine container, combine undrained pineapple, soda pop, half & half, and margarine. Add whole wheat flour, bread flour, Splenda, ginger, nutmeg, and salt. Make an indentation on top of dry ingredients. Pour yeast into indentation. Follow your bread machine's instructions for a 1½-pound loaf. Add coconut and macadamia nuts when "add ingredient" signal beeps. Continue following your machine's instructions. Remove loaf from machine and place on a wire rack to cool. Cut into 12 slices. Makes one (1½-pound) loaf.

Each serving equals:

HE: 1½ Bread • ½ Fat • ¼ Slider • 9 Optional Calories

172 Calories • 4 gm Fat • 5 gm Protein • 29 gm Carbohydrate • 240 mg Sodium • 19 mg Calcium • 2 gm Fiber

DIABETIC EXCHANGES: 1½ Starch • 1 Fat

Barm Brack Bread

I'm so proud of my Irish heritage, and my visit to Ireland a few years ago just confirmed it! This traditional Irish fruit loaf is a baker's classic, eaten on St. Brigid's Feast Day (February 1). Its name comes from words that, translated, mean "speckled bread," and it is often kneaded to a special song. ☻ Serves 12

2 eggs, or equivalent in egg substitute
1 cup unsweetened orange juice
2 tablespoons nonfat dry milk powder
¼ cup reduced-calorie margarine
3 cups bread flour
¼ cup SPLENDA Granular
½ teaspoon ground cinnamon
¼ teaspoon ground nutmeg
¾ teaspoon table salt
1 tablespoon active dry yeast
1 tablespoon candied orange peel, (optional)
½ cup seedless raisins

In a bread-machine container, combine eggs, orange juice, dry milk powder, and margarine. Add bread flour, Splenda, cinnamon, nutmeg, and salt. Make an indentation on top of dry ingredients. Pour yeast into indentation. Follow your bread machine's instructions for a 1½-pound loaf. Add orange peel (if desired) and raisins when "add ingredient" signal beeps. Continue following your machine's instructions. Remove loaf from machine and place on a wire rack to cool. Cut into 12 slices. Makes one (1½-pound) loaf.

Each serving equals:

HE: 1½ Bread • ½ Fruit • ½ Fat • 14 Optional Calories

179 Calories • 3 gm Fat • 6 gm Protein • 32 gm Carbohydrate • 208 mg Sodium • 26 mg Calcium • 1 gm Fiber

DIABETIC EXCHANGES: 1½ Starch • ½ Fat

Marvelous Muffins, Quick Breads, and More

Home bakers have often opted for muffins and quick breads because they're fast and flavorful. Too many store-bought foods in this category are way too high in sugar and fat to be healthy choices, which is another great reason to start (or keep) baking your own sweet sensations! You can even prepare many of these recipes in your toaster oven, if it's big enough for the pan I've called for. Why do it? In warmer seasons, you won't have to heat up your kitchen much—or, if you've assigned other dishes to the oven, you can still enjoy fresh-baked breads and muffins at the same meal.

So dive right in to this collection by stirring up some of my best muffins, cozy winners like *Apricot Chocolate Chip Cheesecake Muffins*, *Carrot and Raisin Muffins*, and *Cliff's Poppy Seed Muffins*. Then spread a little sunshine with some sensational quick breads— *Blueberry Banana Bread*, *Johnny Appleseed Nut Bread*—and some splendid surprises, like *Cherry Kuchen*, *Pecan Pear Scones*, and *Cranberry Coffee Cake Orange Ring*!

Muffin, Quick Bread, and Coffee Cake Baking Tips

You can learn to make breakfast a joyful start to the day, and brunch a festive way to celebrate the weekend—just follow these "best of the best" keys to making speedy sweets!

1. What's the difference between a muffin recipe and a quick bread recipe, you ask? Usually the only difference is what it's baked in, what temperature it's baked at, and for how long. Muffins are baked in muffin tins at higher temperatures for shorter times, while quick breads are baked in loaf pans at lower temperatures for longer times. So if you come across a muffin recipe you'd like to try as a quick bread, lower the temperature to about 350 degrees and bake for 40 to 60 minutes. Likewise, if you'd like to turn a quick bread recipe into muffins, turn the temperature up to 375 to 400 degrees and bake for 12 to 25 minutes (depending on the thickness of the batter).

2. Whether you're making muffins or quick breads, the important thing to remember is to never over-mix the batter. If you mix it too much or too hard, you will overdevelop the gluten in the flour, which will cause your finished product to be tough, with tunnels running through it, and the texture will likely be very compacted. Try to remember to stir only about 10 to 15 times. This is enough to blend the ingredients together and leave the batter still a bit lumpy. Don't worry about those lumps; the batter will continue to blend as it bakes, and the lumps will disappear by the time it is finished baking.

3. Muffin batter should be very soft—not runny and not stiff. If your batter is too thin, sprinkle an extra tablespoon of flour over the batter and stir gently. If your batter is too stiff, add an extra tablespoon or two of the liquid called for in the recipe and stir gently.

4. In most cases, you'll combine the dry ingredients together in one bowl and the wet ingredients together in another bowl. Then quickly blend them together (as per the previous tip). If nuts or fruits are part of the batter, they should be gently stirred in as the last step.

5. Keep an eye on the expiration date on your containers of baking powder and baking soda, and replace them when needed. Your muffins and quick breads will not rise properly if your baking powder or baking soda is old.

6. Be sure that your oven is preheated, and put the muffins and quick breads into the preheated oven as soon as they are poured or spooned into the pan. Batters that use baking powder and baking soda need to be baked immediately so the leavening power is not lost.

7. The best ways to test for doneness in muffins and quick breads: (1) they will spring back when lightly touched; (2) a toothpick will come out clean when inserted near the center; (3) the tops will be lightly browned.

8. To avoid soggy muffins and quick breads, place the baking pan on a wire rack as soon as you remove it from the oven, and cool it in the pan only as long as suggested in the recipe. Remove and continue cooling on a wire rack.

9. Muffins almost always taste best if eaten the same day they are baked. Don't store muffins in the refrigerator; this makes them become stale and dry faster. Keep them covered on the counter for a day or place each muffin (after it's been completely cooled on a wire rack) in an individual Zip-loc freezer bag. Freeze them, and you can have fresh-baked goodness anytime you want. The muffins should keep for up to three months in the freezer.

10. Muffins and quick breads turn out best if baked in the middle of the oven—not near the top or bottom levels, where the temperature can vary by as much as 25 to 30 degrees. If baked on the top rack, the tops brown too soon. If baked on the bottom rack, the bottoms brown

too quickly and may burn. Before you preheat the oven, always check to be sure the rack is in the center; if you do it later, you could burn yourself if you try to change the racks when the oven is already hot!

11. Any muffin cups not used for batter should be filled halfway with water. This helps to ensure even baking of the muffins and protects the pan from warping.

12. Both muffins and slices of quick bread reheat beautifully in the microwave. Place either on a paper plate and cover with a damp paper towel. Heat on HIGH for about 15 to 20 seconds, or just until warm.

Blueberry Orange Muffins

My friend Barbara suggested that these would be a perfect breakfast treat for a New York Knicks or New York Mets fan, as those teams' colors are orange and blue! I told her that no matter who you cheer for, you'll cheer for these!   ☻   Serves 12

> 1¾ cups all-purpose flour
> ½ cup SPLENDA Granular
> 1 tablespoon baking powder
> ½ teaspoon baking soda
> ½ teaspoon table salt
> ½ teaspoon ground cinnamon
> ½ cup fat-free half & half
> ½ cup unsweetened orange juice
> 1 egg, or equivalent in egg substitute
> ¼ cup reduced-calorie margarine
> ¾ cup fresh or frozen blueberries

Preheat oven to 375 degrees. Spray a 12-hole muffin pan with butter-flavored cooking spray, or line with paper liners. In a large bowl, combine flour, Splenda, baking powder, baking soda, salt, and cinnamon. In a medium bowl, combine half & half, orange juice, egg, and margarine. Add liquid mixture to flour mixture. Mix gently just to combine. Gently fold in blueberries. Evenly spoon batter into prepared muffin wells. Bake for 12 to 15 minutes, or until a toothpick inserted in center comes out clean. Place muffin pan on a wire rack and let set for 5 minutes. Remove muffins from pan and continue cooling on wire rack.

HINT: If using frozen blueberries, do not thaw before adding to batter. This will help keep muffins from turning blue.

Each serving equals:

HE: ¾ Bread • ½ Fat • ¼ Slider • 1 Optional Calorie

102 Calories • 2 gm Fat • 3 gm Protein • 18 gm Carbohydrate • 315 mg Sodium • 78 mg Calcium • 1 gm Fiber

DIABETIC EXCHANGES: 1 Starch/Carbohydrate • ½ Fat

Raspberry Muffins

For a special morning, what birthday boy or girl could resist these sweet gems, pretty as they are with ruby fruit "jewels" inside? I wish raspberry season was longer, because the fresh berries produce a slightly better result. But frozen berries are a superb substitute and allow you to enjoy these anytime. ☻ Serves 12

2 cups all-purpose flour
¾ cup SPLENDA Granular
1 tablespoon baking powder
¼ teaspoon table salt
¼ teaspoon ground nutmeg
1 egg, or equivalent in egg
    substitute

½ cup fat-free milk
½ cup fat-free half & half
¼ cup reduced-calorie
    margarine
1½ teaspoons vanilla extract
1 cup fresh or frozen
    raspberries

Preheat oven to 375 degrees. Spray a 12-hole muffin pan with butter-flavored cooking spray, or line with paper liners. In a large bowl, combine flour, Splenda, baking powder, salt, and nutmeg. In a small bowl, combine egg, milk, half & half, margarine, and vanilla extract. Add liquid mixture to flour mixture. Mix gently just to combine. Gently fold in raspberries. Evenly spoon batter into prepared muffin wells. Bake for 20 to 25 minutes, or until a tooth-pick inserted in center comes out clean. Place muffin pan on a wire rack and let set for 5 minutes. Remove muffins from pan and continue cooling on wire rack.

HINT: If using frozen raspberries, do not thaw before adding to batter. This will help keep muffins from turning red.

Each serving equals:

HE: ¾ Bread • ½ Fat • ¼ Slider • 6 Optional Calories

119 Calories • 3 gm Fat • 3 gm Protein • 20 gm Carbohydrate • 219 mg Sodium • 91 mg Calcium • 1 gm Fiber

DIABETIC EXCHANGES: 1 Starch/Carbohydrate • ½ Fat

Heavenly Raspberry Chocolate Chip Muffins

Close your eyes and imagine Fred Astaire and Ginger Rogers dancing to that old classic about being in heaven. Now open them and take a luscious bite of these—why, they're good enough to launch an angelic choir into song! ○ Serves 12

6 tablespoons + 2 teaspoons
  reduced-calorie
  margarine
1¼ cups SPLENDA
  Granular ☆
2 eggs, or equivalent in egg
  substitute
¾ cup fat-free half & half

2 cups all-purpose flour
2 teaspoons baking powder
¼ teaspoon table salt
1½ cups fresh or frozen
  raspberries
¼ cup chopped slivered
  almonds
½ cup mini chocolate chips

Preheat oven to 375 degrees. Spray a 12-hole muffin pan with butter-flavored cooking spray, or line with paper liners. In a large bowl, combine margarine and 1 cup + 2 tablespoons Splenda. Stir in eggs and half & half. In a small bowl, combine flour, baking powder, and salt. Add flour mixture to liquid mixture. Mix gently just to combine. Gently fold in raspberries, almonds, and chocolate chips. Evenly spoon batter into prepared muffin wells. Sprinkle ½ teaspoon Splenda over top of each. Bake for 22 to 26 minutes, or until a toothpick inserted in center comes out clean. Place muffin pan on a wire rack and let set for 5 minutes. Remove muffins from pan and continue cooling on wire rack.

HINT: If using frozen raspberries, do not thaw before adding to batter. This will help keep muffins from turning red.

Each serving equals:

HE: 1 Fat • ¾ Bread • ¼ Protein • ½ Slider • 18 Optional Calories

196 Calories • 8 gm Fat • 5 gm Protein • 26 gm Carbohydrate • 225 mg Sodium • 76 mg Calcium • 2 gm Fiber

DIABETIC EXCHANGES: 1½ Starch/Carbohydrate • 1½ Fat

Oatmeal Cranberry Muffins

Here's a "grab and go" breakfast that tastes yummy fresh out of the oven but freezes beautifully and keeps its sweet and tart flavor when you thaw it for a treat at lunch or a healthy snack.

◐ Serves 8

⅓ cup reduced-calorie margarine
¾ cup SPLENDA Granular
1 egg, or equivalent in egg substitute
½ cup orange juice
1 cup + 2 tablespoons all-purpose flour
½ cup quick oats
1½ teaspoons baking powder
1 teaspoon table salt
1 teaspoon ground cinnamon
1 cup chopped fresh or frozen cranberries

Preheat oven to 375 degrees. Spray 8 wells of a muffin pan with butter-flavored cooking spray, or line with paper liners. In a large bowl, combine margarine, Splenda, and egg, using a wire whisk. Stir in orange juice. In a medium bowl, combine flour, oats, baking powder, salt, and cinnamon. Add flour mixture to liquid mixture. Mix gently just to combine using a sturdy spoon. Gently fold in cranberries. Evenly spoon batter into muffin wells. Bake for 16 to 20 minutes, or until a toothpick inserted in center comes out clean. Place muffin pan on a wire rack and let set for 5 minutes. Remove muffins from pan and continue cooling on wire rack.

Each serving equals:

HE: 1 Bread • 1 Fat • ½ Fruit • 16 Optional Calories

145 Calories • 5 gm Fat • 3 gm Protein • 22 gm Carbohydrate • 465 mg Sodium • 60 mg Calcium • 2 gm Fiber

DIABETIC EXCHANGES: 1 Starch • 1 Fat • ½ Fruit

Banana Cranberry Muffins

This recipe requires more Splenda than some others. Why? Cranberries are extremely tart, more so than many other fruits. In order to enjoy their unique flavor, we need to "super-sweeten" the mix—but the mouthwatering result is well worth it!

◐ Serves 12

2 cups fresh or frozen
    cranberries
1¾ cups SPLENDA
    Granular ☆
1 cup water
⅓ cup reduced-calorie
    margarine
2 eggs, or equivalent in egg
    substitute

1 cup (3 medium) mashed ripe
    bananas
1¾ cups all-purpose flour
2 teaspoons baking powder
¼ teaspoon baking soda
½ teaspoon table salt
½ cup chopped walnuts

Preheat oven to 375 degrees. Spray a 12-hole muffin pan with butter-flavored cooking spray, or line with paper liners. In a medium saucepan, combine cranberries, 1 cup Splenda, and water. Bring mixture to a boil, stirring often. Lower heat and simmer for 6 to 8 minutes, or until cranberries soften, stirring occasionally. Drain cranberries and set aside. In a large bowl, combine margarine, remaining ¾ cup Splenda, and eggs, using a wire whisk. Stir in mashed bananas. In a small bowl, combine flour, baking powder, baking soda, and salt. Add flour mixture to liquid mixture. Mix gently just to combine using a sturdy spoon. Fold in drained cranberries and walnuts. Evenly spoon batter into prepared muffin wells. Bake for 16 to 22 minutes, or until a toothpick inserted in center comes out clean. Place muffin pan on a wire rack and let set for 5 minutes. Remove muffins from pan and continue cooling on wire rack.

Each serving equals:

HE: 1 Fat • ¾ Bread • ⅔ Fruit • ⅓ Protein • 14 Optional Calories

175 Calories • 7 gm Fat • 4 gm Protein • 24 gm Carbohydrate • 262 mg Sodium • 55 mg Calcium • 2 gm Fiber

DIABETIC EXCHANGES: 1 Fat • 1 Starch • ½ Fruit

Carrot and Raisin Muffins

Carrots and raisins each have a special culinary gift to make the other taste even better, don't you think? These fragrant and lush muffins are especially good when served with a little fat-free cream cheese! ● Serves 12

> 2 cups all-purpose flour
> ¾ cup SPLENDA Granular
> 1 tablespoon baking powder
> ¼ teaspoon table salt
> ½ teaspoon apple-pie spice
> ½ cup reduced-calorie margarine
> 2 eggs, or equivalent in egg substitute
> 1 cup fat-free milk
> 1 cup finely shredded carrots
> 1 cup seedless raisins

Preheat oven to 375 degrees. Spray a 12-hole muffin pan with butter-flavored cooking spray or line with paper liners. In a large bowl, combine flour, Splenda, baking powder, salt, and apple-pie spice. In a medium bowl, combine margarine, eggs, and milk. Add liquid mixture to flour mixture. Mix gently just to combine. Fold in carrots and raisins. Evenly spoon batter into prepared muffin wells. Bake for 14 to 18 minutes, or until a toothpick inserted in center comes out clean. Place muffin pan on a wire rack and let set for 5 minutes. Remove muffins from pan and continue cooling on wire rack.

Each serving equals:

HE: 1 Fat • ¾ Bread • ½ Fruit • ¼ Slider • 9 Optional Calories

177 Calories • 5 gm Fat • 4 gm Protein • 29 gm Carbohydrate • 267 mg Sodium • 104 mg Calcium • 1 gm Fiber

DIABETIC EXCHANGES: 1 Fat • 1 Starch • 1 Fruit

Chocolate Peanut Butter Chip Muffins

If there was ever a dynamic duo in the kid-pleasing department, it would have to be chocolate and peanut butter! And some of us never grow up, where this irresistible combo is concerned. . . .

○ Serves 12

½ cup unsweetened applesauce
½ cup quick oats
¼ cup reduced-calorie margarine
1 cup SPLENDA Granular
1 egg, or equivalent in egg substitute
2 tablespoons fat-free half & half
1 teaspoon vanilla extract
¾ cup all-purpose flour
¼ cup unsweetened cocoa powder
1 teaspoon baking powder
½ teaspoon baking soda
½ cup peanut butter chips

Preheat oven to 350 degrees. Spray a 12-hole muffin pan with butter-flavored cooking spray, or line with paper liners. In a medium bowl, combine applesauce and oats. Set aside. In a large bowl, combine margarine, Splenda, egg, half & half, and vanilla extract. Add flour, cocoa powder, baking powder, baking soda, and applesauce mixture. Mix gently just to combine. Fold in peanut butter chips. Evenly spoon batter into prepared muffin wells. Bake for 15 to 20 minutes, or until a toothpick inserted in center comes out clean. Place muffin pan on a wire rack and let set for 5 minutes. Remove muffins from pan and continue cooling on wire rack.

HINTS: 1. If desired, prepare Grandma JO's Chocolate Glaze and drizzle about 1 tablespoon warm glaze over top of each warm muffin.
2. These muffins are very rich, but they do not rise too high.

Each serving equals:

HE: ½ Bread • ½ Fat • ½ Slider • 19 Optional Calories

121 Calories • 5 gm Fat • 3 gm Protein • 16 gm Carbohydrate • 125 mg Sodium • 18 mg Calcium • 2 gm Fiber

DIABETIC EXCHANGES: 1 Starch/Carbohydrate • 1 Fat

Apricot Chocolate Chip Cheesecake Muffins

Can a muffin ever be considered just too good to be true? This one might be a candidate for that award! With its tasty bits of fruit, creamy filling, chocolate bits, and a touch of cinnamon, it's a prizewinner—according to my taste-testers, anyway.

● Serves 12

½ cup reduced-calorie margarine
1 cup + 2 tablespoons SPLENDA Granular ☆
2 eggs, or equivalent in egg substitute
¾ cup fat-free half & half
1½ teaspoons vanilla extract ☆
2 cups all-purpose flour
2 teaspoons baking powder
¼ teaspoon table salt
½ cup finely chopped dried apricots
½ cup fat-free cream cheese
¼ cup mini chocolate chips
½ teaspoon ground cinnamon

Preheat oven to 375 degrees. Spray a 12-hole muffin pan with butter-flavored cooking spray, or line with paper liners. In a large bowl, combine margarine, ¾ cup Splenda, and eggs using a wire whisk. Stir in half & half and 1 teaspoon vanilla extract. In a medium bowl, combine flour, baking powder, and salt. Add flour mixture to liquid mixture. Mix gently just to combine using a sturdy spoon. Fold in apricots. Set aside. In a medium bowl, stir cream cheese with a sturdy spoon until soft. Stir in ¼ cup Splenda, remaining ½ teaspoon vanilla extract, and chocolate chips. Evenly fill muffin wells half full. Drop a full 1 teaspoon cream-cheese filling into center of each. Evenly spoon remaining batter over top of each. In a small bowl, combine remaining 2 tablespoons Splenda, and cinnamon. Evenly sprinkle about ½ teaspoon Splenda/cinnamon mixture over top of each. Bake for 20 to 24 minutes, or until a toothpick inserted in center comes out clean. Place muffin pan on a wire rack and let set for 5 minutes. Remove muffins from pan and continue cooling on wire rack.

Each serving equals:

HE: 1 Fat • ¾ Bread • ⅓ Fruit • ⅓ Protein • ½ Slider • 6 Optional Calories

174 Calories • 6 gm Fat • 5 gm Protein • 25 gm Carbohydrate • 287 mg Sodium • 94 mg Calcium • 2 gm Fiber

DIABETIC EXCHANGES: 1½ Starch/Carbohydrate • 1 Fat • ½ Fruit

Pirate's Pleasure Muffins

Want to be sure you'll never have to walk the plank? Put these on the menu, and any pirates at your house will answer any request with "It would be my pleasure!" They're just that good.

● Serves 12

1 cup nonfat dry milk powder
1¼ cups water
1 tablespoon white distilled vinegar
2¼ cups reduced-fat biscuit baking mix
½ cup SPLENDA Granular
1½ teaspoons baking powder
2 teaspoons reduced-calorie margarine
2 eggs, or equivalent in egg substitute
1½ teaspoons rum extract
¾ cup seedless raisins
¼ cup chopped walnuts

Preheat oven to 375 degrees. Spray a 12-hole muffin pan with butter-flavored cooking spray, or line with paper liners. In a small bowl, combine dry milk powder, water, and vinegar. Let set for 5 minutes. In a large bowl, combine baking mix, Splenda, and baking powder. Add milk mixture, margarine, eggs, and rum extract. Mix gently just to combine. Fold in raisins and walnuts. Evenly spoon batter into prepared muffin wells. Bake for 12 to 16 minutes, or until a toothpick inserted in center comes out clean. Place muffin pan on a wire rack and let set for 5 minutes. Remove scones from pan and continue cooling on wire rack.

Each serving equals:

HE: 1 Bread • ½ Fruit • ¼ Fat-Free Milk • ¼ Protein • ¼ Fat • 4 Optional Calories

164 Calories • 4 gm Fat • 5 gm Protein • 27 gm Carbohydrate • 363 mg Sodium • 140 mg Calcium • 1 gm Fiber

DIABETIC EXCHANGES: 1½ Starch/Carbohydrate • ½ Fruit

Cliff's Poppy Seed Muffins

These are ideal for a take-along snack for any long-distance trucker you happen to know—and they're also perfect to satisfy hungry teens after school! You don't have to squeeze fresh lemons to get the juice, either. Those little plastic lemons filled with juice are just fine. ○ Serves 12

> 2¼ cups all-purpose flour
> 1 cup SPLENDA Granular
> 3 tablespoons poppy seeds
> 2 teaspoons baking powder
> 1 teaspoon baking soda
> ½ teaspoon table salt
> 1 cup plain fat-free yogurt
> ½ cup lemon juice
> 2 eggs, or equivalent in egg substitute
> ¼ cup vegetable oil
> 1½ teaspoons vanilla extract

Preheat oven to 375 degrees. Spray a 12-hole muffin pan with butter-flavored cooking spray, or line with paper liners. In a large bowl, combine flour, Splenda, poppy seeds, baking powder, baking soda, and salt. In a small bowl, combine yogurt, lemon juice, eggs, vegetable oil, and vanilla extract. Add liquid mixture to flour mixture. Mix gently just to combine. Evenly spoon batter into prepared muffin wells. Bake for 18 to 22 minutes, or until a toothpick inserted in center comes out clean. Place muffin pan on a wire rack and let set for 5 minutes. Remove muffins from pan and continue cooling on wire rack.

Each serving equals:

HE: 1 Bread • 1 Fat • ½ Slider • 1 Optional Calorie

175 Calories • 7 gm Fat • 5 gm Protein • 23 gm Carbohydrate • 297 mg Sodium • 120 mg Calcium • 1 gm Fiber

DIABETIC EXCHANGES: 1½ Starch • 1 Fat

Chocolate Chip Eggnog Muffins

If you're not sure what to serve on a holiday morning, I offer you these appealing delights! They've got that unique creamy flavor of everyone's favorite festive beverage, and they can turn an ordinary meal into a feast. Serves 12

½ cup reduced-calorie margarine
1 cup SPLENDA Granular
2 eggs, or equivalent in egg substitute
¾ cup fat-free half & half
1 teaspoon rum extract
2 cups all-purpose flour
2 teaspoons baking powder
1½ teaspoons ground nutmeg
¼ teaspoon table salt
½ cup mini chocolate chips

Preheat oven to 375 degrees. Spray a 12-hole muffin pan with butter-flavored cooking spray, or line with paper liners. In a large bowl, combine margarine, Splenda, and eggs using a wire whisk. Stir in half & half and rum extract. In a small bowl, combine flour, baking powder, nutmeg, and salt. Add flour mixture to liquid mixture. Mix gently just to combine using a sturdy spoon. Fold in chocolate chips. Evenly spoon batter into prepared muffin wells. Bake for 18 to 22 minutes, or until a toothpick inserted in center comes out clean. Place muffin pan on a wire rack and let set for 5 minutes. Remove muffins from pan and continue cooling on wire rack.

Each serving equals:

HE: 1 Fat • ¾ Bread • ¾ Slider • 2 Optional Calories

175 Calories • 7 gm Fat • 4 gm Protein • 24 gm Carbohydrate • 240 mg Sodium • 66 mg Calcium • 1 gm Fiber

DIABETIC EXCHANGES: 1½ Starch/Carbohydrate • 1 Fat

Blueberry Banana Bread

You'll never feel "blue" when you're dining on a slice of this beautiful bread that brims over with berries and sweet banana bits! It packs well for school lunches and offers real health benefits, too.

● Serves 8

> ¾ cup SPLENDA Granular
> ¼ cup reduced-calorie margarine
> 1 egg, or equivalent in egg substitute
> ⅔ cup (2 medium) mashed ripe bananas
> ¼ cup fat-free half & half
> 1 teaspoon vanilla extract
> 1½ cups all-purpose flour
> ½ teaspoon baking soda
> ½ teaspoon table salt
> ¾ cup fresh or frozen blueberries

Preheat oven to 350 degrees. Spray a 9-by-5-inch loaf pan with butter-flavored cooking spray. In a large bowl, combine Splenda and margarine. Stir in egg and bananas. Add half & half and vanilla extract. Mix well to combine. Add flour, baking soda, and salt. Mix gently just to combine. Gently fold in blueberries. Evenly spread batter into prepared loaf pan. Bake for 50 to 60 minutes, or until a toothpick inserted in center comes out clean. Place loaf pan on a wire rack and let set for 10 minutes. Remove bread from pan and continue cooling on wire rack. Cut into 8 slices.

HINT: If using frozen blueberries, do not thaw before adding to batter. This will help keep bread from turning blue.

Each serving equals:

HE: 1 Bread • ¾ Fat • ⅔ Fruit • ¼ Slider • 1 Optional Calorie

160 Calories • 4 gm Fat • 4 gm Protein • 27 gm Carbohydrate • 312 mg Sodium • 17 mg Calcium • 2 gm Fiber

DIABETIC EXCHANGES: 1 Starch • 1 Fat • ½ Fruit

Mom's Peanut Butter Quick Bread

Do your kids love peanut butter as much as mine always did? I decided to create a lip-smacking good quick bread that's as much fun to eat as a peanut-butter-and-jelly sandwich! It's ready fast, and makes a fun after-school snack. ☻ Serves 8

> 1 cup + 2 tablespoons all-purpose flour
> ½ cup quick oats
> ¾ cup SPLENDA Granular
> 1 tablespoon baking powder
> ½ teaspoon table salt
> 1 cup fat-free milk
> ¼ cup fat-free half & half
> 1 egg, or equivalent in egg substitute
> ½ cup reduced-fat chunky peanut butter

Preheat oven to 350 degrees. Spray a 9-by-5-inch loaf pan with butter-flavored cooking spray. In a large bowl, combine flour, oats, Splenda, baking powder, and salt. Add milk, half & half, egg, and peanut butter. Mix gently just to combine. Evenly spread batter into prepared loaf pan. Bake for 55 to 60 minutes, or until a toothpick inserted in center comes out clean. Place loaf pan on a wire rack and let set for 10 minutes. Remove bread from pan and continue cooling on wire rack. Cut into 8 slices.

Each serving equals:

HE: 1 Bread • 1 Protein • 1 Fat • ¼ Slider • 4 Optional Calories

211 Calories • 7 gm Fat • 9 gm Protein • 28 gm Carbohydrate • 438 mg Sodium • 144 mg Calcium • 2 gm Fiber

DIABETIC EXCHANGES: 1½ Starch/Carbohydrate • 1 Meat • ½ Fat

Johnny Appleseed Nut Bread

I've doubled the flavor and fun in this fruit and nut bread by adding both applesauce and apple juice to the batter! When you stir in some apple-pie spice, you'll want to hang around your own kitchen because it smells so good. ☻ Serves 8

¼ cup reduced-calorie margarine
1 cup SPLENDA Granular
1 egg, or equivalent in egg substitute
2 tablespoons unsweetened apple juice
½ cup unsweetened applesauce
1¼ cups reduced-fat biscuit baking mix
¼ cup graham cracker crumbs
1 teaspoon apple-pie spice
2 teaspoons baking powder
¼ teaspoon table salt
¼ cup chopped walnuts

Preheat oven to 350 degrees. Spray a 9-by-5-inch loaf pan with butter-flavored cooking spray. In a large bowl, combine margarine, Splenda, and egg, using a wire whisk. Stir in apple juice and applesauce. In another large bowl, combine baking mix, graham cracker crumbs, apple-pie spice, baking powder, and salt. Add baking mix mixture to liquid mixture. Mix gently just to combine, using a sturdy spoon. Fold in walnuts. Evenly spread batter into prepared loaf pan. Bake for 40 to 45 minutes, or until a toothpick inserted in center comes out clean. Place loaf pan on a wire rack and let set for 10 minutes. Remove bread from pan and continue cooling on wire rack. Cut into 8 slices.

Each serving equals:

HE: 1 Bread • 1 Fat • ¼ Protein • 19 Optional Calories

159 Calories • 7 gm Fat • 3 gm Protein • 21 gm Carbohydrate • 483 mg Sodium • 87 mg Calcium • 1 gm Fiber

DIABETIC EXCHANGES: 1 Starch • 1 Fat

Zucchini Raisin Nut Bread

Let me assure you that zucchini bread doesn't taste like a bowl of veggies—I promise! Some real kitchen magic occurs when you shred the zukes into this bread batter. The result is nothing short of fantastic! ◐ Serves 8

¾ cup SPLENDA Granular
¼ cup reduced-calorie margarine
1 egg, or equivalent in egg substitute
¼ cup unsweetened applesauce
1 teaspoon vanilla extract
1½ cups all-purpose flour
2 teaspoons baking powder
½ teaspoon ground cinnamon
½ teaspoon table salt
1 cup shredded zucchini
½ cup seedless raisins
¼ cup chopped walnuts

Preheat oven to 350 degrees. Spray a 9-by-5-inch loaf pan with butter-flavored cooking spray. In a large bowl, combine Splenda, margarine, and egg using a wire whisk. Stir in applesauce and vanilla extract. Add flour, baking powder, cinnamon, and salt. Mix gently just to combine, using a sturdy spoon. Fold in zucchini, raisins, and walnuts. Evenly spread batter into prepared loaf pan. Bake for 40 to 46 minutes, or until a toothpick inserted in center comes out clean. Place loaf pan on a wire rack and let set for 10 minutes. Remove bread from pan and continue cooling on wire rack. Cut into 8 slices.

Each serving equals:

HE: 1 Bread • 1 Fat • ½ Fruit • ¼ Protein • ¼ Vegetable • 12 Optional Calories

186 Calories • 6 gm Fat • 4 gm Protein • 29 gm Carbohydrate • 325 mg Sodium • 80 mg Calcium • 2 gm Fiber

DIABETIC EXCHANGES: 1 Starch • 1 Fat • 1 Fruit

Banana Chocolate Chip Quick Bread

Nature packs loads of potassium into each bright-yellow banana, delivering great nutrition and sweet flavor in every bite. I love baking with bananas, because they seem to sparkle even brighter when they spend some time in a hot oven. Enjoy!   ☻   Serves 8

¼ cup reduced-calorie margarine
¼ cup unsweetened applesauce
1 cup SPLENDA Granular
2 eggs, or equivalent in egg substitute
1 cup (3 medium) mashed ripe bananas
1 teaspoon vanilla extract
1½ cups all-purpose flour
1 teaspoon baking soda
⅛ teaspoon table salt
¼ cup mini chocolate chips
¼ cup chopped walnuts

Preheat oven to 350 degrees. Spray a 9-by-5-inch loaf pan with butter-flavored cooking spray. In a large bowl, combine margarine, applesauce, Splenda, and eggs, using a wire whisk. Stir in mashed bananas and vanilla extract. Add flour, baking soda, and salt. Mix gently just to combine, using a sturdy spoon. Fold in chocolate chips and walnuts. Evenly spread batter into prepared loaf pan. Bake for 50 to 60 minutes, or until a toothpick inserted in center comes out clean. Place loaf pan on a wire rack and let set for 10 minutes. Remove bread from pan and continue cooling on wire rack. Cut into 8 slices.

Each serving equals:

HE: 1 Bread • 1 Fat • ¾ Fruit • ⅓ Protein • ¼ Slider • 11 Optional Calories

220 Calories • 8 gm Fat • 5 gm Protein • 32 gm Carbohydrate • 281 mg Sodium • 19 mg Calcium • 2 gm Fiber

DIABETIC EXCHANGES: 1 Starch • 1 Fat • 1 Fruit

Pumpkin Chocolate Chip Holiday Quick Bread

One of a cook's best kitchen tricks is keeping a quick bread moist and delicious. A terrific ingredient to ensure that? Canned pumpkin! It's available year-round, it's inexpensive, and it blends beautifully with other flavors (like chocolate!).

○ Makes 2 loaves; Serves 16

⅔ cup reduced-calorie margarine
3 cups SPLENDA Granular
3 eggs, or equivalent in egg substitute
1 (15-ounce) can solid-pack pumpkin
1½ teaspoons vanilla extract
3 cups all-purpose flour
1 tablespoon pumpkin-pie spice
1 tablespoon baking powder
1 teaspoon baking soda
½ teaspoon table salt
½ cup mini chocolate chips

Preheat oven to 350 degrees. Spray two 9-by-5-inch loaf pans with butter-flavored cooking spray. In a large bowl, combine margarine, SPLENDA, and eggs using a wire whisk. Stir in pumpkin and vanilla extract. Add flour, pumpkin-pie spice, baking powder, baking soda, and salt. Mix gently just to combine using a sturdy spoon. Fold in chocolate chips. Evenly spread batter into prepared loaf pans. Bake for 44 to 48 minutes, or until a toothpick inserted in center comes out clean. Place loaf pans on a wire rack and let set for 10 minutes. Remove bread from pans and continue cooling on wire rack. When serving, cut each loaf into 8 slices.

Each serving equals:

HE: 1 Bread • 1 Fat • ¼ Vegetable • ½ Slider • 12 Optional Calories

199 Calories • 6 gm Fat • 4 gm Protein • 28 gm Carbohydrate • 296 mg Sodium • 64 mg Calcium • 2 gm Fiber

DIABETIC EXCHANGES: 2 Starch/Carbohydrate • 1 Fat

Cherry Kuchen

Some of our most beloved food memories are gifts from our ancestors, recipes that immigrants carried here with them many years ago. This cozy, sweet bread is one of my son James's favorite tastes of childhood—and today, he shares it with his three sons!

♥ Serves 8

1½ cups + 4 tablespoons all-purpose flour ☆
¾ cup SPLENDA Granular ☆
2 teaspoons baking powder
⅓ cup reduced-calorie margarine ☆

2 eggs, or equivalent in egg substitute
⅓ cup fat-free half & half
1 teaspoon vanilla extract
1 (20-ounce) can sugar-free cherry pie filling
¼ teaspoon ground cinnamon

Preheat oven to 350 degrees. Spray an 8-by-8-inch baking dish with butter-flavored cooking spray. In a large bowl, combine ½ cups flour, ½ cup Splenda, and baking powder. Add ¼ cup margarine, eggs, half & half, and vanilla extract. Mix gently just to combine. Evenly spread batter into prepared baking dish. Bake for 15 minutes. Spoon cherry pie filling evenly over partially baked kuchen. In a small bowl, combine remaining 4 tablespoons flour, remaining ¼ cup Splenda, cinnamon, and remaining 1 tablespoon + 1 teaspoon margarine. Mix well using a pastry blender or 2 forks until mixture becomes crumbly. Evenly sprinkle crumb topping over cherry pie filling. Continue baking for 10 to 15 minutes. Place pan on a wire rack and let set for 30 minutes. Cut into 8 servings.

HINT: If you can't find purchased sugar-free cherry pie filling, use Grandma JO's Pie Filling.

Each serving equals:

HE: 1 Bread • 1 Fat • ½ Fruit • ¼ Protein • ¼ Slider • 8 Optional Calories

185 Calories • 5 gm Fat • 5 gm Protein • 30 gm Carbohydrate • 230 mg Sodium • 82 mg Calcium • 2 gm Fiber

DIABETIC EXCHANGES: 1½ Starch • 1 Fat • ½ Fruit

Cranberry Coffee Cake Orange Ring

There's something so impressive about serving a homemade coffee cake ring—and you get to take all the credit! What more inviting brunch finale could you offer your in-laws some Sunday?

◑ Serves 12

> 2 cups all-purpose flour
> 1 cup SPLENDA Granular
> 1½ teaspoons baking powder
> ½ teaspoon baking soda
> ½ teaspoon table salt
> ¼ teaspoon apple-pie spice
> ¾ cup unsweetened orange juice
> 1 egg, or equivalent in egg substitute
> 2 tablespoons vegetable oil
> 1 teaspoon vanilla extract
> 1 cup whole fresh or frozen cranberries

Preheat oven to 350 degrees. Spray a Bundt pan with butter-flavored cooking spray. In a large bowl, combine flour, Splenda, baking powder, baking soda, salt, and apple-pie spice. In a small bowl, combine orange juice, egg, vegetable oil, and vanilla extract. Add liquid mixture to flour mixture. Mix gently just to combine, using a sturdy spoon. Fold in cranberries. Evenly spread batter into prepared pan. Bake for 28 to 36 minutes, or until a toothpick inserted in center comes out clean. Place pan on a wire rack and let set for 15 minutes. Gently loosen coffee cake from pan with a knife. Invert onto a serving plate and allow to cool completely. Cut into 12 servings.

Each serving equals:

HE: ¾ Bread • ½ Fat • ¼ Slider • 4 Optional Calories

119 Calories • 3 gm Fat • 3 gm Protein • 20 gm Carbohydrate • 206 mg Sodium • 38 mg Calcium • 1 gm Fiber

DIABETIC EXCHANGES: 1 Starch • ½ Fat

Cranberry Streusel Coffee Cake

It's been such fun to take old-fashioned baking recipes and transform them into twenty-first-century "delectables"! Making your own coffee cake from scratch may seem a bit overwhelming, but it's much easier than you ever expected. 😊 Serves 8

> 1 egg, or equivalent in egg substitute
> ¾ cup SPLENDA Granular ☆
> ½ cup fat-free half & half
> 1 tablespoon vegetable oil
> 1 tablespoon unsweetened orange juice
> ¼ teaspoon vanilla extract
> 1½ cups all-purpose flour ☆
> 2 teaspoons baking powder
> ½ teaspoon table salt
> 2 cups chopped fresh or frozen cranberries
> 2 tablespoons reduced-calorie margarine

Preheat oven to 350 degrees. Spray an 8-by-8-inch baking dish with butter-flavored cooking spray. In a large bowl, beat egg until fluffy using a wire whisk. Add ½ cup Splenda, half & half, vegetable oil, orange juice, and vanilla extract. Mix gently just to combine. Stir in 1 cup flour, baking powder, and salt. Evenly spread batter into prepared baking dish. Spoon cranberries evenly over batter. In a small bowl, combine remaining ½ cup flour and remaining ¼ cup Splenda. Add margarine. Mix well using a pastry blender or 2 forks until mixture becomes crumbly. Evenly sprinkle crumb mixture over cranberries. Bake for 20 to 30 minutes. Place baking dish on a wire rack and let set for 5 minutes. Cut into 8 servings. Serve warm.

Each serving equals:

HE: 1 Bread • ¾ Fat • ¼ Fruit • ¼ Slider • 6 Optional Calories

152 Calories • 4 gm Fat • 4 gm Protein • 25 gm Carbohydrate • 310 mg Sodium • 84 mg Calcium • 2 gm Fiber

DIABETIC EXCHANGES: 1½ Starch/Carbohydrate • 1 Fat

Lemon Poppy Seed Bundt Coffee Cake

If you loaned your Bundt pan to your daughter-in-law (and never asked for it back), this recipe will provide an excellent reason to reclaim it! The pairing of lemon with poppy seeds is a delicate flavor duet that works astonishingly well. ❍ Serves 12

1 cup SPLENDA Granular
½ cup reduced-calorie margarine
2 eggs, or equivalent in egg substitute
½ cup fat-free half & half
¼ cup lemon juice
1½ teaspoons vanilla extract
2 cups cake flour
2 teaspoons baking powder
¼ teaspoon table salt
2 tablespoons poppy seeds

Preheat oven to 350 degrees. Spray a Bundt pan with butter-flavored cooking spray. In a large bowl, combine Splenda, margarine, and eggs. Mix with an electric mixer on LOW until well blended. Stir in half & half, lemon juice, and vanilla extract. Add flour, baking powder, salt, and poppy seeds. Continue beating on LOW for 2 minutes, or until batter is smooth. Evenly spread batter into prepared pan. Bake for 30 minutes, or until a toothpick inserted in center comes out clean. Place pan on a wire rack and let set for 5 minutes. Gently loosen cake from pan with a knife. Invert onto a serving plate and allow to cool completely. Cut into 12 servings.

HINT: If desired, lightly dust with Grandma JO's Powdered Sugar.

Each serving equals:

HE: 1 Fat • ¾ Bread • ½ Slider • 2 Optional Calories

129 Calories • 5 gm Fat • 3 gm Protein • 18 gm Carbohydrate • 232 mg Sodium • 79 mg Calcium • 1 gm Fiber

DIABETIC EXCHANGES: 1 Starch • 1 Fat

Luscious Lemon
Pound Cake Loaf

I hope the recipe title makes my feelings clear: I'm thrilled to have created a traditional lemon pound cake that is low in fat and uses the marvelous magic of Splenda to make it oh-so-sweet!

● Serves 8

⅓ cup reduced-calorie margarine
1 cup SPLENDA Granular
2 eggs, or equivalent in egg substitute
½ cup fat-free sour cream
¼ cup lemon juice

1½ cups all-purpose flour
1 teaspoon baking powder
½ teaspoon baking soda
¼ teaspoon table salt
1 to 2 tablespoons grated lemon peel, optional

Preheat oven to 325 degrees. Spray a 9-by-5-inch loaf pan with butter-flavored cooking spray. In a large bowl, combine margarine and Splenda, using a wire whisk. Stir in eggs, sour cream, and lemon juice. Add flour, baking powder, baking soda, and salt. Mix gently just to combine using a sturdy spoon. Fold in lemon peel, if desired. Evenly spread batter into prepared loaf pan. Bake for 55 to 65 minutes, or until a toothpick inserted in center comes out clean. Place loaf pan on a wire rack and let set for 10 minutes. Remove bread from pan and continue cooling on wire rack. Cut into 8 slices.

HINTS: 1. This loaf does not raise as high as usual.
2. If desired, turn this into a dessert by spooning Grandma JO's Lemon Sauce over top.

Each serving equals:

HE: 1 Bread • 1 Fat • ¼ Protein • ¼ Slider • 7 Optional Calories

161 Calories • 5 gm Fat • 5 gm Protein • 24 gm Carbohydrate • 329 mg Sodium • 63 mg Calcium • 1 gm Fiber

DIABETIC EXCHANGES: 1½ Starch • 1 Fat

Pecan Pear Scones

Even though we took our country back from the British in 1776, they left us with a few memorable culinary prizes—including a passion for scones! Now you can prepare your own version at home, including this fruit-and-nut variety. ☺ Serves 8

½ cup SPLENDA Granular
¼ cup reduced-calorie margarine
1 egg, or equivalent in egg substitute
½ cup fat-free half & half
2 tablespoons fat-free sour cream
1½ cups all-purpose flour
2 teaspoons baking powder
¼ teaspoon table salt
1 cup (2 small) chopped peeled pears
2 tablespoons chopped pecans

Preheat oven to 375 degrees. Spray a baking sheet with butter-flavored cooking spray. In a large bowl, combine Splenda, margarine, and egg using a wire whisk. Stir in half & half and sour cream. Add flour, baking powder, and salt. Mix well to combine using a sturdy spoon. Fold in pears and pecans. Drop mixture by large tablespoonful to form 8 scones. Bake for 14 to 18 minutes, or until golden brown. Lightly spray top of scones with butter-flavored cooking spray. Remove scones from baking sheet and place on a wire rack. Serve warm.

Each serving equals:

HE: 1 Bread • 1 Fat • ¼ Fruit • ¼ Slider • 8 Optional Calories

165 Calories • 5 gm Fat • 4 gm Protein • 26 gm Carbohydrate • 276 mg Sodium • 91 mg Calcium • 2 gm Fiber

DIABETIC EXCHANGES: 1½ Starch/Carbohydrate • 1 Fat

Grandma's
Baking Powder Biscuits

Even if your grandma used her oven to store her old tax returns, you can make scrumptious biscuits that taste like a grandma made them! These are easy and delightful, ready in a jiffy, and sure to please a crowd. ☻ Serves 8

> 1½ cups + 2 tablespoons cake flour ☆
> 2 tablespoons SPLENDA Granular
> 1 tablespoon baking powder
> ½ teaspoon table salt
> ¼ cup reduced-calorie margarine
> ½ cup fat-free half & half

Preheat oven to 425 degrees. In a large bowl, combine 1½ cups flour, Splenda, baking powder, and salt. Add margarine. Mix well using a pastry blender or 2 forks until mixture resembles fine crumbs. Add half & half. Using a sturdy spoon, mix just until mixture makes a soft, easy-to-roll dough. Sprinkle remaining 2 tablespoons flour on a clean counter and shape dough into a ball on floured counter. Pat mixture into a large circle. Using a 2-inch biscuit cutter, form into 8 biscuits, patting dough together as necessary. Place biscuits on an ungreased baking sheet. Prick each biscuit several times with the tines of a fork. Lightly spray tops with butter-flavored cooking spray. Bake for 10 to 12 minutes, or until golden brown. Serve hot.

Each serving equals:

HE: 1 Bread • ¾ Fat • 10 Optional Calories

111 Calories • 3 gm Fat • 2 gm Protein • 19 gm Carbohydrate • 385 mg Sodium • 109 mg Calcium • 1 gm Fiber

DIABETIC EXCHANGES: 1 Starch • 1 Fat

Chocolate Chip Cranberry Drop Biscuits

A drop biscuit differs from the traditional kind because, instead of rolling out the dough and cutting out squares, it asks you to drop the dough onto the baking sheets instead of cutting out individual biscuits. Now you can serve these and be relaxed when company comes for brunch!   ☻   Serves 6

> ¾ cup reduced-fat biscuit baking mix
> ¼ cup + 1 tablespoon SPLENDA Granular ☆
> 1 teaspoon baking powder
> ¼ cup fat-free half & half
> 1 tablespoon fat-free sour cream
> ¼ cup dried cranberries or craisins
> 2 tablespoons mini chocolate chips

Preheat oven to 375 degrees. Spray a baking sheet with butter-flavored cooking spray. In a large bowl, combine baking mix, ¼ cup Splenda, and baking powder. Add half & half and sour cream. Mix gently just to combine. Fold in cranberries and chocolate chips. Drop batter onto prepared baking sheet to form 6 biscuits. Lightly spray tops with butter-flavored cooking spray. Sprinkle ½ teaspoon Splenda over top of each. Bake for 12 to 16 minutes, or until light golden brown. Place baking sheet on a wire rack and let set for 5 minutes. Serve warm.

Each serving equals:

HE: ⅔ **Bread** • ⅓ **Fruit** • ¼ **Slider** • 10 **Optional Calories**

102 Calories • 2 gm Fat • 2 gm Protein • 19 gm Carbohydrate • 259 mg Sodium • 69 mg Calcium • 1 gm Fiber

DIABETIC EXCHANGES: 1 Starch/Carbohydrate

Creamy Cakes

I t's such fun to feel confident about baking your own special-occasion cakes—and to have a bundle of dazzlers to choose from when it's time to preheat the oven and bake up a storm! Cakes are one of the first well-loved foods many people give up when they find out they've got diabetes or high cholesterol, but it's no fun to sit at the table in front of an empty dessert plate because you're worried about your health. Instead, take the initiative and make a cake that you know you can enjoy without fear—and if you've been invited somewhere for a party, bring something along to share with others who may also have the same concerns!

They've always been popular for children's birthdays, but these days, cupcakes are showing up at everything from office lunches to weddings. So why not whip up a batch of *Cappuccino Cupcakes* for a card party or some *Pretty Pink Peppermint Cupcakes* for a holiday-season bridal shower? For a taste of sunny climes, try *Island Sun Cake* or *Lime Poke Cake*. And to show your family that lovin' does sometimes come from the oven, mix up *Applesauce Raisin Rum Cake* or *Cherry Angel Food Cake Roll*!

Cake-Baking Cooking Tips

Want to bake a perfect cake every time? Of course you do! Here's all the advice you'll need to make every cake a masterpiece. Once you know these kitchen secrets, you'll be ready to stir up every recipe in this chapter—and any other cake recipe that sounds good.

1. One of the most important "secrets" to being a good cake baker is measuring carefully. What does that mean? All measurements should be as perfectly level as possible. All dry ingredients should be measured in measuring cups,

the ones that come four different sizes to a set. But liquid ingredients should be measured in a liquid measuring cup. And don't guess with the tiny amounts—measuring spoons are a must.

If you don't already have good standard measuring equipment in your kitchen, invest in some before starting to bake, especially cakes! My measuring cups have the amounts printed on the handles in bold lettering, so I don't have to squint while trying to read them. I have both 1-cup and 2-cup liquid measuring cups in my cupboard, with the amounts printed in bright red. As soon as they've been washed so often that it becomes hard to read them, I replace them. My measuring spoons also have the amounts printed on the handles. I separated them from the ring that held them together so that it's easier to use only the one I need. I just keep them stored together in an organizer in my cupboard.

2. Other equipment I consider important to successful cake baking: a wire whisk, sturdy mixing spoons, quality rubber spatulas, and metal cooling racks. (Make sure your rack can hold a minimum of a dozen cookies.) Just as a good carpenter has his toolbox equipped with the right tools, it's important to have your kitchen stocked with the right kitchen tools for the task at hand.

3. You can use either regular butter-flavored cooking spray or the flour-coating cooking spray when preparing your cake pans. I prefer the flour-coating kind, but when I run out and I want to make a cake, the regular works just fine.

4. If the recipe calls for a 9-by-9-inch cake pan and all you have is an 8-by-8-inch baking dish, don't panic! You can usually substitute your pan—but only IF you remember to lower the oven temperature by 25 degrees OR shorten the baking time by about 10 to 15 minutes. Either should work, but don't do both.

5. Always preheat the oven. Turn the oven on to the suggested temperature before you start gathering your equip-

ment and ingredients to make the cake. This allows plenty of time to get the oven up to the required temperature. Also, before you turn the oven on, check the racks to see that they are at or near the middle of the oven, where the heat is most likely to be the most even.

6. If your cakes seem to bake too quickly, or if they just never seem to get done in the center, it might be that your oven's actual temperature is different from what the setting says. Invest in a good oven thermometer. You might be surprised to learn that your oven is baking 75 or more degrees hotter or colder than you thought it was! Once you know your oven's true temperature, you can either have your oven repaired or learn to use the oven thermometer as your gauge instead of the oven setting.

7. Always test your cake for doneness at the minimum time suggested in the recipe. Here are the two easiest ways I know to test if a cake is done: (1) Insert a cake tester or toothpick into the center of the cake. If the cake it done, the tester will come out clean. (2) Touch the cake lightly with a finger. If the cake springs back, leaving no imprint, then the cake is done. If either test shows that the cake is not done, bake it a few minutes longer, then test it again. Whichever method you choose, remember not to open the oven door until the minimum baking time has arrived, and *never* shift the pans around during baking. Both are sure to cause "cake failure"!

8. With very few exceptions, cakes should be thoroughly cooled before you slice or frost them. For proper cooling, the air should be able to circulate freely around all sides of the cake. That's why my directions always include placing the cake pan on a wire rack. This allows the cake to cool quickly and evenly.

9. Because sponge cakes and angel food cakes have such an extremely fragile structure, they must "hang" upside down while cooling. To do this, as soon as you take one of these cakes from the oven, *immediately* turn it upside

down and let it cool for about 2 hours. If it is fully baked, it will not fall out, since the pan has not been greased or treated in any way. The tube pans used for these kinds of cakes have a tube through the center that extends above the rim of the pan. The inverted cake may rest on this inner tube, to allow air to circulate. Sometimes the pans have side "ears," which they rest on when turned upside down. If your tube pan has neither an extended center tube nor the "ears," rest the tube over a narrow-necked bottle or inverted funnel. When the cake has cooled (at least 2 hours) turn it right side up, insert a spatula or narrow knife between the cake and the edge of the pan, and lift the cake out. Then turn the cake so it's right side up.

10. Egg whites, for angel food or sponge cakes, beat up lighter and more easily if they are at room temperature. They should be neither too warm nor too cold. The best advice is to remove the eggs from the refrigerator and let them sit on the counter at room temperature for two or three hours before they are beaten. Also, never place eggs in a metal pan when whipping them. Always use a large glass bowl.

11. While some of my snack cake recipes may call for all-purpose flour, most of my cake recipes call for cake flour. Why? It has less protein than all-purpose flour and gives the cakes a finer crumb and a softer texture. But be sure to read the labels in the store carefully, so that you *don't* buy "self-rising" cake flour by accident. This product has baking powder added and could throw off the chemistry of your batter just enough so that your cake won't turn out correctly. The flour you use really does make a difference. What if you're out of cake flour? In such an "emergency," you can make 1 cup of cake flour by combining ¾ cup of all-purpose flour and 2 tablespoons of cornstarch.

12. While testing recipes for this book, I discovered that in almost all cases, combining the margarine and Splenda

with a wire whisk before blending in the other liquid ingredients makes for a better cake. After the flour and other dry ingredients are added, a long, sturdy spoon works best to mix the batter. And a rubber spatula is what I use to evenly spread the batter into the prepared pan. It scrapes out every bit of batter from the bowl and makes wash-up a snap!

Easy Cupcakes

These are my "no excuses, ever," anyone-can-make-'em party pleasers. Even first-time bakers can really shine when they bring these to the table. ● Serves 8

> ½ cup reduced-calorie margarine
> 2 tablespoons unsweetened applesauce
> 1 cup SPLENDA Granular
> 2 eggs, or equivalent in egg substitute
> ½ cup fat-free half & half
> 1 teaspoon vanilla extract
> 1½ cups cake flour
> 1½ teaspoons baking powder

Preheat oven to 350 degrees. Line 8 muffin wells with paper liners. In a large bowl, combine margarine, applesauce, and Splenda using a wire whisk. Stir in eggs, half & half, and vanilla extract. Add flour and baking powder. Mix gently just to combine using a sturdy spoon. Evenly spoon batter into prepared muffin wells. Bake for 14 to 18 minutes, or until a toothpick inserted in center comes out clean. Place muffin pan on a wire rack and let set for 5 minutes. Remove cupcakes and cool on wire rack.

HINTS: 1. Fill unused muffin wells with water. It protects the muffin tin and ensures even baking.
2. If desired, frost with Grandma JO's Chocolate Glaze, Grandma JO's Peanut Butter Glaze, or Grandma JO's Butter Cream Frosting.

Each serving equals:

HE: 1 Bread • 1 Fat • ¼ Protein • ¼ Slider • 2 Optional Calories

145 Calories • 5 gm Fat • 4 gm Protein • 21 gm Carbohydrate • 204 mg Sodium • 71 mg Calcium • 1 gm Fiber

DIABETIC EXCHANGES: 1 Starch/Carbohydrate • 1 Fat

Cappuccino Cupcakes

Did you know that cupcakes are often selected by brides and grooms as a more "fun" alternative to "boring" wedding cakes? It's true. But if you want to be sure your treats are for mature audiences, why not try these velvety darlings? ● Serves 8

¼ cup reduced-calorie margarine
¾ cup SPLENDA Granular
2 eggs, or equivalent in egg substitute
⅔ cup cold coffee
1½ teaspoons vanilla extract
1½ cups reduced-fat biscuit baking mix
¼ cup unsweetened cocoa powder
½ teaspoon ground cinnamon

Preheat oven to 350 degrees. Line 8 muffin wells with paper liners. In a large bowl, combine margarine, Splenda, and eggs using a wire whisk. Stir in coffee and vanilla extract. In a small bowl, combine baking mix, cocoa powder, and cinnamon. Add baking mix mixture to margarine mixture. Mix gently just to combine using a sturdy spoon. Spoon batter half full into prepared muffin wells. Bake for 18 to 20 minutes, or until a toothpick inserted in center comes out clean. Place muffin pan on a wire rack and let set for 5 minutes. Remove cupcakes and cool on wire rack.

HINT: Frost with Grandma JO's Chocolate Glaze if desired.

Each serving equals:

HE: 1 Bread • ¾ Fat • ¼ Protein • 15 Optional Calories

150 Calories • 6 gm Fat • 4 gm Protein • 20 gm Carbohydrate • 348 mg Sodium • 34 mg Calcium • 1 gm Fiber

DIABETIC EXCHANGES: 1½ Starch/Carbohydrate • 1 Fat

Pretty Pink Peppermint Cupcakes

It's not only young ladies who love to be pretty in pink—sometimes, it's cupcakes, too! These are perfect party fare for a birthday, a tea party, or a special sleepover. ☻ Serves 8

> 2 tablespoons + 2 teaspoons reduced-calorie margarine
> ¾ cup SPLENDA Granular
> 2 eggs, or equivalent in egg substitute
> ⅔ cup fat-free milk
> ¼ teaspoon peppermint extract
> 3 to 4 drops red food coloring
> 1½ cups reduced-fat biscuit baking mix
> ¼ cup crushed sugar-free peppermint candies

Preheat oven to 350 degrees. Line 8 muffin wells with paper liners. In a large bowl, combine margarine, Splenda, and eggs using a wire whisk. Stir in milk, peppermint extract, and red food coloring. Add baking mix and peppermint candies. Mix gently just to combine using a sturdy spoon. Spoon batter half full into prepared muffin wells. Bake for 18 to 22 minutes, or until a toothpick inserted in center comes out clean. Place muffin pan on a wire rack and let set for 5 minutes. Remove cupcakes and cool on wire rack.

Each serving equals:

HE: 1 Bread • ½ Fat • ¼ Protein • ¼ Slider • 6 Optional Calories

136 Calories • 4 gm Fat • 4 gm Protein • 21 gm Carbohydrate • 333 mg Sodium • 54 mg Calcium • 1 gm Fiber

DIABETIC EXCHANGES: 1½ Starch/Carbohydrate • ½ Fat

Angel Food Cupcakes

Light and airy, these heavenly delights are a lovely end to a hearty meal, when everyone worries about having room for dessert. No one's too full to enjoy a fluffy cupcake like this one!

◔ Serves 6

6 egg whites
1 teaspoon cream of tartar
¼ teaspoon table salt
1 teaspoon vanilla extract
¾ cup SPLENDA Granular
½ cup + 1 tablespoon cake flour

Preheat oven to 375 degrees. Line 6 muffin wells with paper liners. Place egg whites in a very large glass mixing bowl. Beat egg whites with an electric mixer on HIGH until foamy. Add cream of tartar, salt, and vanilla extract. Continue beating until stiff enough to form soft peaks. Add Splenda, ¼ cup at a time, while continuing to beat egg whites until stiff peaks form. Fold in cake flour using a spatula or wire whisk. Evenly spoon batter into prepared muffin wells. Bake for 14 to 16 minutes, or until cakes spring back when lightly touched. Place muffin pan on a wire rack and let set for 5 minutes. Remove cupcakes and cool on wire rack.

HINT: If desired, frost with Grandma JO's Chocolate Glaze or top with Grandma JO's Heavenly Fruit Topping.

Each serving equals:

HE: ½ Bread • ¼ Protein • 12 Optional Calories

68 Calories • 0 gm Fat • 5 gm Protein • 12 gm Carbohydrate • 153 mg Sodium • 4 mg Calcium • 0 gm Fiber

DIABETIC EXCHANGES: 1 Starch

Surprise Cupcakes

Just when your family members think they know what's for dessert, surprise them with these mouth-watering mystery munchies! The filling is unexpected but never unwelcome. Enjoy!

● Serves 12

1½ cups cake flour
1½ cups SPLENDA
    Granular ☆
¼ cup unsweetened cocoa
    powder
1 teaspoon baking soda
½ teaspoon table salt
1 cup water
1 tablespoon + 1 teaspoon
    reduced-calorie margarine
¼ cup reduced-fat peanut
    butter

1 tablespoon white distilled
    vinegar
1½ teaspoons vanilla extract
1 (8-ounce) package fat-free
    cream cheese
1 egg, or equivalent in egg
    substitute
¼ cup mini chocolate chips
¼ cup peanut butter chips,
    chopped

Preheat oven to 350 degrees. Line 12 muffin wells with paper liners. In a large bowl, combine flour, 1 cup Splenda, cocoa powder, baking soda, and salt. Add water, margarine, peanut butter, vinegar, and vanilla extract. Mix well to combine. Evenly spoon batter into prepared muffin wells, filling each half full. In a medium bowl, stir cream cheese with a sturdy spoon until softened. Add egg and remaining ½ cup Splenda. Mix well to combine. Fold in chocolate chips and peanut butter chips. Evenly spoon a full 1 tablespoon cream cheese mixture over top of each cupcake. Bake for 20 to 25 minutes. Place muffin pan on a wire rack and let set for 5 minutes. Remove cupcakes and cool on wire rack.

Each serving equals:

HE: ¾ Protein • ⅔ Bread • ½ Fat • ½ Slider • 12 Optional Calories

170 Calories • 6 gm Fat • 7 gm Protein • 22 gm Carbohydrate • 218 mg Sodium • 65 mg Calcium • 2 gm Fiber

DIABETIC EXCHANGES: 1½ Starch/Carbohydrate • ½ Meat • ½ Fat

Cherry Angel Food Cake Roll

This gorgeous "jelly roll" looks special enough to have come from a bakery, but you can make it at home with fresh and luscious ingredients! The colorful cherries peeking out of each slice are temptation all by themselves.   ♥   Serves 8

1 cup cake flour	2 tablespoons vanilla extract
1½ cups SPLENDA	¼ teaspoon table salt
Granular ☆	1 (20-ounce) can sugar-free
12 egg whites	cherry pie filling

Preheat oven to 350 degrees. Line a 15½-by-10½-by-1-inch jelly-roll pan with either parchment paper or waxed paper. In a small bowl, combine cake flour and ¾ cup Splenda. Mix well using a wire whisk. Place egg whites in a very large glass mixing bowl. Beat egg whites with an electric mixer on HIGH until foamy. Add vanilla extract and salt. Continue beating until stiff enough to form soft peaks. Add remaining ¾ cup Splenda, 2 tablespoons at a time, while continuing to beat egg whites until stiff peaks form. Add the flour mixture, ½ cup at a time, folding in with spatula or wire whisk. Evenly spread batter into prepared pan. Bake for 12 to 15 minutes, or until cake is set. Place a clean cotton dish towel on counter and immediately invert cake onto towel. Carefully remove paper. Roll up cake with towel, in jelly-roll fashion, starting at short end. Allow to cool completely. Unroll cake and remove towel. Spread pie filling to within 1 inch of edges of cake. Re-roll and place on serving plate, seam side down. Refrigerate for at least 30 minutes. Cut into 8 servings.

HINT: If desired, lightly dust with Grandma JO's Powdered Sugar, drizzle with Grandma JO's Chocolate Glaze, or garnish each piece with a dollop of reduced-calorie whipped topping.

Each serving equals:

HE: ⅔ Bread • ½ Protein • ½ Fruit • 18 Optional Calories

120 Calories • 0 gm Fat • 7 gm Protein • 23 gm Carbohydrate • 164 mg Sodium • 5 mg Calcium • 1 gm Fiber

DIABETIC EXCHANGES: 1 Starch/Other Carbohydrate • ½ Meat

Lime Poke Cake

I love a cake with a secret, don't you? This is a delectable cake all by itself, but as I like to say, good enough isn't good enough for me. So I invite you to perform a little culinary magic, which might make other cooks at the table green with envy! ☻ Serves 12

¼ cup reduced-calorie margarine
1 cup SPLENDA Granular
2 eggs, or equivalent in egg substitute
1 cup fat-free milk
1½ teaspoons vanilla extract
2 cups reduced-fat biscuit baking mix

1 (4-serving) package sugar-free lime gelatin
1 cup boiling water
½ cup cold water
2 cups reduced-calorie whipped topping
green sugar crystals, optional

Preheat oven to 350 degrees. Spray a 9-by-13-inch cake pan with butter-flavored cooking spray. In a large bowl, combine margarine, Splenda, and eggs, using a wire whisk. Stir in milk and vanilla extract. Add baking mix. Mix gently just to combine using a sturdy spoon. Spread batter evenly into prepared pan. Bake for 18 to 22 minutes, or until a toothpick inserted in the center comes out clean. Place pan on a wire rack and let set for 15 minutes. In a medium bowl, combine dry gelatin and boiling water. Mix well to dissolve gelatin, using a wire whisk. Stir in cold water. Pierce cake with a large fork at ½-inch intervals. Carefully pour gelatin mixture over cake. Refrigerate for 2 hours. Evenly spread whipped topping over top of cake. If desired, lightly sprinkle green sugar crystals over top. Refrigerate for at least 1 hour. Cut into 12 servings.

HINT: Use any flavor gelatin and any color sugar crystals.

Each serving equals:

HE: ¾ Bread • ½ Fat • ½ Slider • 19 Optional Calories

141 Calories • 5 gm Fat • 4 gm Protein • 20 gm Carbohydrate • 318 mg Sodium • 51 mg Calcium • 1 gm Fiber

DIABETIC EXCHANGES: 1½ Starch/Carbohydrate • ½ Fat

Strawberry Dream Cake

My kitchen helpers know without asking which cake I'd choose to serve for my birthday: this sensational strawberry cake that's a dream-come-true in every bite! It's impressive to look at, and even better to taste. ☻ Serves 8

2 tablespoons + 2 teaspoons reduced-calorie margarine
¾ cup SPLENDA Granular ☆
1 egg, or equivalent in egg substitute
2 tablespoons fat-free sour cream
½ cup fat-free milk

1 tablespoon vanilla extract
1 cup + 2 tablespoons reduced-fat biscuit baking mix
2 cups frozen unsweetened strawberries, completely thawed and undrained
1½ cups reduced-calorie whipped topping

Preheat oven to 350 degrees. Spray a 9-by-9-inch cake pan with butter-flavored cooking spray. In a large bowl, combine margarine and ½ cup Splenda using a wire whisk. Stir in egg, sour cream, milk, and vanilla extract. Add baking mix. Mix gently just to combine using a sturdy spoon. Evenly spread batter into prepared cake pan. Bake for 16 to 20 minutes, or until a toothpick inserted in the center comes out clean. Do not overbake. Place pan on a wire rack and allow to cool for 30 minutes. Poke holes 1-inch apart on top of cake using the handle of a wooden spoon. In a blender container, combine undrained strawberries and remaining ¼ cup Splenda. Cover and process on BLEND for 30 seconds, or until mixture is smooth. Reserve ⅓ cup blended mixture. Evenly spread remaining blended strawberry mixture over cooled cake. Refrigerate for 30 minutes. In a medium bowl, gently combine whipped topping and reserved strawberry mixture. Evenly spread over top. Refrigerate for at least 30 minutes. Cut into 8 servings.

Each serving equals:

HE: ¾ Bread • ½ Fat • ¼ Fruit • ½ Slider • 17 Optional Calories

149 Calories • 5 gm Fat • 3 gm Protein • 23 gm Carbohydrate • 262 mg Sodium • 54 mg Calcium • 1 gm Fiber

DIABETIC EXCHANGES: 1½ Starch/Carbohydrate • ½ Fat

Easy Sponge Cake

I'll confess that even an easy sponge cake does ask you to separate a few eggs, but that's always been easier than you may have thought! Once your yolks and whites are placed in different bowls, this cake is surprisingly easy to make—and wonderfully satisfying to serve.

❂ Serves 8

> 6 egg whites
> 4 egg yolks
> 1 cup SPLENDA Granular ☆
> 1 cup + 2 tablespoons cake flour
> 1 teaspoon baking powder
> ½ teaspoon vanilla extract

Preheat oven to 325 degrees. In a large bowl, beat egg whites with an electric mixer on HIGH until stiff peaks form. In a medium bowl, beat egg yolks with a wire whisk until fluffy. Stir ½ cup Splenda into egg whites. Stir remaining ½ cup Splenda into egg yolks. Carefully stir egg-yolk mixture into egg-white mixture using a wire whisk. Add flour and baking powder. Mix gently just to combine, using a wire whisk. Stir in vanilla extract. Evenly spread batter into an ungreased metal angel food cake pan. Bake for 35 to 40 minutes, or until a toothpick inserted in center comes out clean. Invert cake in pan on a funnel or bottle neck. Allow to cool completely, about 1½ hours. Gently loosen cake from pan with a table knife. Place serving plate on top of pan and gently shake cake loose. Cut into 8 servings.

HINT: An ungreased 9-by-13-inch metal cake pan can be used instead of an angel food cake pan.

Each serving equals:

HE: ¾ Bread • ½ Protein • 12 Optional Calories

123 Calories • 3 gm Fat • 6 gm Protein • 18 gm Carbohydrate • 96 mg Sodium • 45 mg Calcium • 0 gm Fiber

DIABETIC EXCHANGES: 1 Starch • ½ Meat

Orange Glow Bundt Cake

Whether you're a morning person or an evening person, whether that beautiful warm light you see in the sky is sunrise or sunset, this is an amazing cake to add to your repertoire. It's lip-smacking yummy, rich in flavor, and oh so pretty when it's "unmolded" onto the serving plate. ☻ Serves 12

> ¼ cup reduced-calorie margarine
> 1½ cups SPLENDA Granular ☆
> 2 eggs, or equivalent in egg substitute
> 1½ cups unsweetened orange juice ☆
> ½ cup diet lemon-lime soda pop
> 2 teaspoons coconut extract ☆
> 2 cups reduced-fat biscuit baking mix
> 2 tablespoons cornstarch
> 3 tablespoons flaked coconut

Preheat oven to 350 degrees. Spray a Bundt pan with butter-flavored cooking spray. In a large bowl, combine margarine, 1 cup Splenda, and eggs using a wire whisk. Stir in ½ cup orange juice, soda pop, and 1½ teaspoons coconut extract. Add baking mix. Mix gently just to combine using a sturdy spoon. Evenly spread batter into prepared pan. Bake for 30 minutes, or until a toothpick inserted in the center comes out clean. Place pan on a wire rack and let set for 15 minutes. Gently loosen cake from pan with a knife and turn out onto wire rack. Meanwhile, in a medium saucepan, combine cornstarch, remaining ½ cup Splenda, and remaining 1 cup orange juice. Cook over medium heat until mixture thickens and starts to boil, stirring constantly with a wire whisk. Remove from heat. Stir in remaining ½ teaspoon coconut extract. Let set for 5 minutes. Place cooled cake on a serving plate and evenly drizzle orange sauce over cake. Evenly sprinkle coconut over top. Refrigerate for at least 30 minutes. Cut into 12 servings.

Each serving equals:

HE: ¾ Bread • ½ Fat • ¼ Fruit • ¼ Slider • 8 Optional Calories

136 Calories • 4 gm Fat • 3 gm Protein • 22 gm Carbohydrate • 294 mg Sodium • 28 mg Calcium • 1 gm Fiber

DIABETIC EXCHANGES: 1½ Starch • ½ Fat

Coconut Chocolate Chip Bundt Cake

While I don't think *everything* is better in a Bundt pan, I do love to present attractive cakes I've baked in this popular shape. This recipe teaches chocolate and coconut to tango together in a truly splendid dance of flavors. Light a few candles, put on some music, and you'll be ready to dance when dinner's done!

● Serves 16

⅔ cup reduced-calorie margarine
2 cups SPLENDA Granular
3 eggs, or equivalent in egg substitute
½ cup (4-ounces) fat-free cream cheese, softened
⅓ cup unsweetened applesauce
1 teaspoon vanilla extract
1¼ cups fat-free half & half
2 teaspoons coconut extract
3 cups cake flour
½ teaspoon baking soda
¼ teaspoon table salt
½ cup flaked coconut
½ cup mini chocolate chips

Preheat oven to 325 degrees. Spray a Bundt pan with butter-flavored cooking spray. In a large bowl, combine margarine, Splenda, and eggs using a wire whisk. Stir in softened cream cheese, applesauce, and vanilla extract using a wire whisk. Add half & half and coconut extract. Mix well with a sturdy spoon until softened. In a medium bowl, combine flour, baking soda, and salt. Add flour mixture to margarine mixture. Mix gently just to combine using a sturdy spoon. Fold in coconut and chocolate chips. Evenly spread batter into prepared pan. Bake for 50 to 60 minutes, or until a toothpick inserted in center comes out clean. Place pan on a wire rack and let set for 15 minutes. Gently loosen cake from pan with a knife and invert onto a serving plate. Let set for at least 30 minutes. Cut into 16 servings.

HINTS: 1. This is a very heavy, moist cake.

2. If desired, lightly dust with Grandma JO's Powdered Sugar.

Each serving equals:

HE: 1 Bread • 1 Fat • ⅓ Protein • ¾ Slider • 1 Optional Calorie

187 Calories • 7 gm Fat • 5 gm Protein • 26 gm Carbohydrate • 247 mg Sodium • 50 mg Calcium • 1 gm Fiber

DIABETIC EXCHANGES: 2 Starch/Carbohydrate • 1 Fat

Chocolate Swirl Cake

There's something so sensual and satisfying about a cake that beckons you to enjoy a piece of its curvy, chocolate center! This tender cake is a terrific party choice, but you don't need a special occasion to mix it up. ◑ Serves 12

½ cup fat-free half & half
½ cup fat-free milk
1 tablespoon white distilled vinegar
½ cup reduced-calorie margarine
1½ cups SPLENDA Granular
3 eggs, or equivalent in egg substitute
½ cup unsweetened applesauce
1½ teaspoons coconut extract
2¼ cups reduced-fat biscuit baking mix
1¼ teaspoons baking soda ☆
½ teaspoon table salt
½ cup flaked coconut
½ cup reduced-calorie chocolate syrup

Preheat oven to 350 degrees. Spray a Bundt pan with butter-flavored cooking spray. In a small bowl, combine half & half, milk, and vinegar. Set aside. In a large bowl, combine margarine, Splenda, and eggs using a wire whisk. Stir in applesauce, milk mixture, and coconut extract. In a small bowl, combine baking mix, 1 teaspoon baking soda, salt, and coconut. Add baking mix mixture to margarine mixture. Mix gently just to combine using a sturdy spoon. Measure 2 cups of the batter and place in a medium bowl. Stir in chocolate syrup and remaining ¼ teaspoon baking soda. Evenly pour remaining batter into prepared Bundt pan. Drizzle chocolate batter evenly over top. Do Not Mix. Bake for 50 to 60 minutes, or until a toothpick inserted in center comes out clean. Place pan on a wire rack and let set for 15 minutes. Gently loosen cake from pan with a knife and invert onto a serving plate. Let set for at least 30 minutes. Cut into 12 servings.

HINT: If desired, prepare Grandma JO's Chocolate Glaze and drizzle over top of cooled cake.

Each serving equals:

HE: 1 Bread • 1 Fat • ¼ Protein • ¾ Slider • 7 Optional Calories

203 Calories • 7 gm Fat • 5 gm Protein • 30 gm Carbohydrate • 635 mg Sodium • 60 mg Calcium • 1 gm Fiber

DIABETIC EXCHANGES: 2 Starch/Carbohydrate • 1 Fat

Chocolate Cream Layer Cake

As the song says, "I'm old-fashioned," and I love the romantic things in life, like this luscious layer cake! It takes a few extra minutes to assemble this oh-so-excellent prizewinner, but it's time well spent. ◐ Serves 12

⅓ cup reduced-calorie margarine
1½ cups SPLENDA Granular ☆
2 eggs, or equivalent in egg substitute
¼ cup fat-free sour cream
1 cup fat-free half & half
6 tablespoons reduced-calorie chocolate syrup ☆
1 tablespoon vanilla extract ☆
¼ cup unsweetened cocoa powder
2 cups reduced-fat biscuit baking mix
1 teaspoon baking powder
1 (8-ounce) package fat-free cream cheese
2 cups reduced-calorie whipped topping
¼ cup finely chopped pecans ☆

Preheat oven to 350 degrees. Spray two (9-inch) round cake pans with butter-flavored cooking spray. In a large bowl, combine margarine and 1 cup Splenda using a wire whisk. Stir in eggs, sour cream, half & half, 2 tablespoons chocolate syrup, and 2 teaspoons vanilla extract. Blend in cocoa. (Batter will be lumpy.) Add baking mix and baking powder. Mix gently just to combine using a sturdy spoon. Evenly spread batter into prepared cake pans. Bake for 18 to 22 minutes, or until a toothpick inserted in the center comes out clean. Place pans on wire racks and let set for 10 minutes. Remove cakes from pans and continue cooling on wire racks. In a large bowl, stir cream cheese with a sturdy spoon until softened. Add whipped topping and remaining 1 teaspoon vanilla extract. Mix gently just to combine using a wire whisk. Fold in remaining ¼ cup chocolate syrup. Place 1 cake on a serving plate. Spread ⅓ of mixture over cake. Sprinkle 2 tablespoons pecans over top. Arrange remaining cake over filling. Spread remaining filling over top and on sides of cake. Evenly sprinkle remaining 2 tablespoons pecans over top. Refrigerate for at least 30 minutes. Cut into 12 servings.

HINT: If you prefer, you can split each cake to make four layers, spread ¼ of filling over each layer, and turn this cake into a torte.

Each serving equals:

HE: 1 Fat • ¾ Bread • ½ Protein • ¾ Slider • 18 Optional Calories

212 Calories • 8 gm Fat • 7 gm Protein • 28 gm Carbohydrate • 496 mg Sodium • 162 mg Calcium • 1 gm Fiber

DIABETIC EXCHANGES: 1½ Starch/Carbohydrate • 1 Fat • ½ Meat

Classic Chocolate Cake

Ideal for all kinds of occasions, this recipe's a baker's dream. Its texture is velvety, its flavor magnificent—and its appeal timeless.

⚫ Serves 12

> ½ cup reduced-calorie margarine
> 1½ cups SPLENDA Granular
> 1 cup fat-free milk
> ½ cup fat-free half & half
> 2 eggs, or equivalent in egg substitute
> 1 teaspoon vanilla extract
> 2¼ cups cake flour
> ½ cup unsweetened cocoa powder
> 1 teaspoon baking powder
> 1 teaspoon baking soda

Preheat oven to 350 degrees. Spray a 9-by-13-inch cake pan with butter-flavored cooking spray. In a large bowl, combine margarine and Splenda using a wire whisk. Stir in milk, half & half, eggs, and vanilla extract. In a small bowl, combine flour, cocoa powder, baking powder, and baking soda. Add flour mixture to margarine mixture. Mix gently to combine using a sturdy spoon. Evenly spread batter into prepared cake pan. Bake for 14 to 18 minutes, or until a toothpick inserted in center comes out clean. Place pan on a wire rack and allow to cool completely. Cut into 12 servings.

Each serving equals:

HE: 1 Bread • 1 Fat • ¼ Slider • 17 Optional Calories

153 Calories • 5 gm Fat • 4 gm Protein • 23 gm Carbohydrate • 265 mg Sodium • 68 mg Calcium • 1 gm Fiber

DIABETIC EXCHANGES: 1½ Starch • 1 Fat

Choca-Cola Cake

I've been teased for liking to cook and bake with soda pop, but I just smile and say, "Taste it before you decide it's a funny idea." Cola has been a beloved cake flavoring since soon after it came onto the market all those years ago, and it's still yummy today!

🌣 Serves 12

½ cup reduced-calorie
   margarine
1¾ cups SPLENDA Granular
2 eggs, or equivalent in egg
   substitute
2 tablespoons fat-free sour
   cream

2 teaspoons vanilla extract
1½ cups diet cola soda pop
2¼ cups reduced-fat biscuit
   baking mix
¼ cup unsweetened cocoa
   powder
1 teaspoon baking powder

Preheat oven to 350 degrees. Spray a 9-by-13-inch cake pan with butter-flavored cooking spray. In a large bowl, combine margarine and Splenda using a wire whisk. Stir in eggs, sour cream, vanilla extract, and soda pop. Add baking mix, cocoa powder, and baking powder. Mix gently just to combine using a sturdy spoon. Evenly spread batter into prepared cake pan. Bake for 22 to 26 minutes, or until a toothpick inserted in center comes out clean. Place pan on a wire rack and allow to cool completely. Cut into 12 servings.

HINTS: 1. Good topped with 2 recipes of Grandma JO's Chocolate Glaze if desired.
2. Also good topped with a dollop of reduced-calorie whipped topping. If using don't forget to count the additional calories.

Each serving equals:

HE: 1 Bread • 1 Fat • ¼ Slider • 1 Optional Calorie

154 Calories • 6 gm Fat • 4 gm Protein • 21 gm Carbohydrate • 401 mg Sodium • 54 mg Calcium • 1 gm Fiber

DIABETIC EXCHANGES: 1½ Starch/Carbohydrate • 1 Fat

Mocha Fudge Cake

No, this cake wasn't inspired by one of my friend Barbara's favorite ice creams, but she's not alone in loving the combo of coffee and luxurious fudge. Try serving this when friends stop by to admire your garden or your grandkids!   ❤   Serves 8

¾ cup cold coffee
1 cup SPLENDA Granular
1 teaspoon vanilla extract
⅓ cup reduced-calorie margarine
1 cup + 2 tablespoons cake flour
¼ cup unsweetened cocoa powder
½ teaspoon baking powder
½ teaspoon baking soda
¼ teaspoon table salt

Preheat oven to 350 degrees. Spray a 9-inch round cake pan with butter-flavored cooking spray. In a large bowl, combine coffee, Splenda, vanilla extract, and margarine. Mix well using a wire whisk. Add flour, cocoa powder, baking powder, baking soda, and salt. Mix gently to combine using a sturdy spoon. Evenly spread batter into prepared cake pan. Bake for 14 to 16 minutes, or until a toothpick inserted in center comes out clean. Do not overbake. Place pan on a wire rack and allow to cool completely. Cut into 8 servings.

HINTS: 1. This is a flat, moist cake that doesn't rise very much.
2. If desired, top with either Grandma JO's Raspberry Sauce or Grandma JO's Fudge Glaze.

Each serving equals:

HE: 1 Fat • ¾ Bread • 18 Optional Calories

108 Calories • 4 gm Fat • 2 gm Protein • 16 gm Carbohydrate • 267 mg Sodium • 22 mg Calcium • 1 gm Fiber

DIABETIC EXCHANGES: 1 Starch • 1 Fat

Chocolate Zucchini Spice Cake

You may have to take it on faith that you can make an appealing chocolate cake with that very green vegetable—but you truly can! This is a really moist cake that also delivers the bonus of a little extra fiber along with tasty flavor. ☻ Serves 8

>2 tablespoons + 2 teaspoons reduced-calorie margarine
>1 egg, or equivalent in egg substitute
>¾ cup Splenda Granular
>⅔ cup fat-free half & half
>1½ teaspoons vanilla extract
>1½ cups reduced-fat biscuit baking mix
>2 tablespoons unsweetened cocoa powder
>1½ teaspoons apple-pie spice
>1 teaspoon baking powder
>¼ teaspoon table salt
>1 cup finely shredded unpeeled zucchini
>¼ cup chopped walnuts

Preheat oven to 350 degrees. Spray a 9-by-9-inch cake pan with butter-flavored cooking spray. In a large bowl, combine margarine, egg, Splenda, half & half, and vanilla extract. Mix well using a wire whisk. Add baking mix, cocoa powder, apple-pie spice, baking powder, and salt. Mix gently just to combine using a sturdy spoon. Fold in zucchini and walnuts. Evenly spread batter into prepared cake pan. Bake for 18 to 22 minutes, or until a toothpick inserted in center comes out clean. Place pan on a wire rack and allow to cool completely. Cut into 8 servings.

HINT: If desired, frost with Grandma JO's Chocolate Glaze.

Each serving equals:

HE: 1 Bread • ¾ Fat • ¼ Protein • ¼ Vegetable • ¼ Slider • 3 Optional Calories

167 Calories • 7 gm Fat • 4 gm Protein • 22 gm Carbohydrate • 396 mg Sodium • 86 mg Calcium • 1 gm Fiber

DIABETIC EXCHANGES: 1½ Starch/Carbohydrate • 1 Fat

Roundup Time Spice Cake

The inspiration for this cake comes from all the way back in the 1950s, when a clever cook stirred a can of tomato soup into her cake batter. The result was so good, a cake "fad" was born, and I've decided to celebrate her ingenuity with this updated version!

❂ Serves 8

> 2 tablespoons + 2 teaspoons reduced-calorie margarine
> ¾ cup SPLENDA Granular
> 1 (10¾-ounce) can reduced-fat tomato soup
> 2 tablespoons fat-free sour cream
> 1 tablespoon fat-free half & half
> 1½ teaspoons pumpkin-pie spice
> 1½ cups cake flour
> 1 teaspoon baking soda
> ½ teaspoon baking powder
> ¾ cup seedless raisins

Preheat oven to 350 degrees. Spray a 9-by-9-inch cake pan with butter-flavored cooking spray. In a large bowl, combine margarine and Splenda using a wire whisk. Stir in tomato soup, sour cream, half & half, and pumpkin-pie spice. In a small bowl, combine flour, baking soda, and baking powder. Add flour mixture to margarine mixture. Mix gently just to combine using a sturdy spoon. Fold in raisins. Spread batter evenly into prepared pan. Bake for 18 to 24 minutes, or until a toothpick inserted in center comes out clean. Place pan on a wire rack and allow to cool completely. Cut into 8 servings.

HINT: Good served with a dollop of reduced-calorie whipped topping. If using, don't forget to count the additional calories.

Each serving equals:

HE: 1 Bread • ¾ Fruit • ¾ Fat • ½ Slider • 1 Optional Calorie

175 Calories • 3 gm Fat • 2 gm Protein • 35 gm Carbohydrate • 379 mg Sodium • 34 mg Calcium • 1 gm Fiber

DIABETIC EXCHANGES: 1½ Starch/Other Carbohydrate • 1 Fruit • 1 Fat

Cheyanne's Fruit Cocktail Cake

Is there a child who doesn't adore that old classic, canned fruit cocktail? (If there is, he or she isn't one of my grandkids!) I've dedicated this recipe to one of my darling granddaughters, who loves helping in the kitchen, especially when cake is on the menu!

⟲ Serves 8

¼ cup reduced-calorie
   margarine
¾ cup SPLENDA Granular
1 egg, or equivalent in egg
   substitute
1 (15-ounce) can fruit cocktail,
   packed in fruit juice,
   undrained
1 teaspoon coconut extract

1⅓ cups cake flour
1 teaspoon baking powder
1 teaspoon baking soda
½ teaspoon table salt
¼ cup chopped walnuts
2 tablespoons graham-cracker
   crumbs
2 tablespoons flaked coconut

Preheat oven to 350 degrees. Spray a 9-by-9-inch cake pan with butter-flavored cooking spray. In a large bowl, combine margarine, Splenda, and egg using a wire whisk. Stir in undrained fruit cocktail and coconut extract. In a small bowl, combine flour, baking powder, baking soda, and salt. Add flour mixture to margarine mixture. Mix gently just to combine using a sturdy spoon. Stir in walnuts. Evenly spread batter into prepared cake pan. In a small bowl, combine graham-cracker crumbs and coconut. Sprinkle crumb mixture evenly over top. Bake for 23 to 25 minutes, or until a toothpick inserted in center comes out clean. Place pan on a wire rack and allow to cool completely. Cut into 8 servings.

HINT: Good served with a dollop of reduced-calorie whipped topping. If using, don't forget to count the additional calories.

Each serving equals:

HE: 1 Bread • 1 Fat • ½ Fruit • ¼ Protein • 14 Optional Calories

166 Calories • 6 gm Fat • 3 gm Protein • 25 gm Carbohydrate • 443 mg Sodium • 45 mg Calcium • 1 gm Fiber

DIABETIC EXCHANGES: 1 Starch • 1 Fat • ½ Fruit

Country Carrot Cake

While this is certainly one way to get your kids to eat a few more carrots, this dessert isn't beloved because it's good for you—it's just plain old wonderful on its own merits. It's good the day it comes out of the oven, and I think it's even better a few days (or even weeks, if you freeze it) later. ☯ Serves 8

¼ cup reduced-calorie margarine
¾ cup SPLENDA Granular
3 eggs, or equivalent in egg substitute
1 cup fat-free half & half
1½ teaspoons vanilla extract
1½ cups reduced-fat biscuit baking mix
1½ teaspoons ground cinnamon
2 cups grated carrots
¼ cup chopped walnuts

Preheat oven to 350 degrees. Spray a 9-by-9-inch cake pan with butter-flavored cooking spray. In a large bowl, combine margarine, Splenda, and eggs using a wire whisk. Stir in half & half and vanilla extract. Add baking mix and cinnamon. Mix well to combine using a sturdy spoon. Stir in carrots and walnuts. Evenly spread batter into prepared pan. Bake for 33 to 37 minutes, or until a toothpick inserted in center comes out clean. Place pan on a wire rack and allow to cool completely. Cut into 8 servings.

HINTS: 1. If desired, lightly dust with Grandma JO's Powdered Sugar.
2. Also good topped with a dollop of reduced-calorie whipped topping.
   If using, don't forget to count the additional calories.

Each serving equals:

HE: 1 Bread • 1 Fat • ½ Protein • ½ Vegetable • ¼ Slider • 7 Optional Calories

201 Calories • 9 gm Fat • 6 gm Protein • 24 gm Carbohydrate • 418 mg Sodium • 79 mg Calcium • 2 gm Fiber

DIABETIC EXCHANGES: 1 Starch • 1 Fat • ½ Meat • ½ Vegetable

Island Sun Cake

What a lovely thought in the deep, dark months of winter to imagine lying on a beach in the Caribbean or Hawaii, soaking up all that vitamin D the sun delivers in every ray! But sometimes sun comes wrapped in a sweetly seductive dessert like this one. Put away the sunscreen and pick up a fork!   ☻   Serves 8

¼ cup reduced-calorie margarine
½ cup SPLENDA Granular
2 (8-ounce) cans crushed pineapple, packed in fruit juice,
    undrained
3 tablespoons fat-free half & half
1 teaspoon coconut extract
1½ cups cake flour
1 teaspoon baking powder
½ teaspoon baking soda
¼ cup flaked coconut
2 tablespoons chopped pecans

Preheat oven to 350 degrees. Spray a 9-by-9-inch cake pan with butter-flavored cooking spray. In a large bowl, combine margarine and Splenda using a wire whisk. Stir in undrained pineapple, half & half, and coconut extract. In a small bowl, combine flour, baking powder, and baking soda. Add flour mixture to margarine mixture. Mix gently just to combine using a sturdy spoon. Fold in coconut and pecans. Evenly spread batter into prepared cake pan. Bake for 30 to 40 minutes, or until a toothpick inserted in center comes out clean. Place pan on a wire rack and allow to cool completely. Cut into 8 servings.

Each serving equals:

HE: 1 Bread • 1 Fat • ½ Fruit • 19 Optional Calories

169 Calories • 5 gm Fat • 2 gm Protein • 29 gm Carbohydrate • 212 mg Sodium • 50 mg Calcium • 1 gm Fiber

DIABETIC EXCHANGES: 1 Starch • 1 Fat • ½ Fruit

Scrumptious Banana Cake

Don't toss out those blackened bananas—bake up a storm! Ripe bananas give a basic cake batter an incredible sweetness, and this simple recipe is a great choice for brunch or supper, or just an after-school snack.   ♥   Serves 8

2 tablespoons + 2 teaspoons reduced-calorie margarine
¾ cup SPLENDA Granular
2 eggs, or equivalent in egg substitute
⅔ cup (2 medium) mashed ripe bananas
½ cup water
1½ teaspoons vanilla extract
1½ cups reduced-fat biscuit baking mix

Preheat oven to 350 degrees. Spray a 9-by-9-inch cake pan with butter-flavored cooking spray. In a large bowl, combine margarine, Splenda, and eggs using a wire whisk. Stir in mashed bananas, water, and vanilla extract. Add baking mix. Mix gently just to combine using a sturdy spoon. Evenly spread batter into prepared cake pan. Bake for 20 to 24 minutes, or until a toothpick inserted in center comes out clean. Place pan on a wire rack and allow to cool completely. Cut into 8 servings.

HINT: If desired, frost with Grandma JO's Chocolate Glaze.

Each serving equals:

HE: 1 Bread • ½ Fruit • ½ Fat • ¼ Protein • 9 Optional Calories

149 Calories • 5 gm Fat • 4 gm Protein • 22 gm Carbohydrate • 324 mg Sodium • 31 mg Calcium • 1 gm Fiber

DIABETIC EXCHANGES: 1 Starch • ½ Fruit • ½ Fat

Applesauce Raisin Rum Cake

It's nutty, fruity, and just a little naughty—no, I'm kidding, rum extract isn't really alcoholic!—but it tastes so sinfully good, you might worry that this cake will tempt you off the straight-and-narrow path! I'm so sure it's okay, I've served it for Sunday lunch after church. 🌑 Serves 12

¼ cup chopped pecans
½ cup reduced-calorie margarine
1 cup SPLENDA Granular
1½ cups unsweetened applesauce
1 tablespoon rum extract
2¼ cups cake flour
2 teaspoons apple-pie spice
1 cup + 2 tablespoons seedless raisins
1 tablespoon hot water
2 teaspoons baking soda

Preheat oven to 325 degrees. Spray a Bundt pan with butter-flavored cooking spray. Evenly sprinkle pecans over bottom of prepared pan. In a large bowl, combine margarine and Splenda using a wire whisk. Stir in applesauce and rum extract. Add flour, apple-pie spice, and raisins. Mix well to combine using a sturdy spoon. In a small bowl, combine hot water and baking soda. Gently stir mixture into batter. Evenly spread batter into prepared pan. Bake for 45 to 55 minutes, or until a toothpick inserted in center comes out clean. Place pan on a wire rack and let set for 15 minutes. Gently loosen cake from pan with a knife and invert onto a serving plate. Let set for at least 30 minutes. Cut into 12 servings.

Each serving equals:

HE: 1 Bread • 1 Fruit • 1 Fat • 8 Optional Calories

190 Calories • 6 gm Fat • 2 gm Protein • 32 gm Carbohydrate • 303 mg Sodium • 17 mg Calcium • 2 gm Fiber

DIABETIC EXCHANGES: 1 Starch • 1 Fruit • 1 Fat

Black Walnut Cake

If you're lucky enough to live next to a walnut tree, you already know how spectacular a cake starring this well-loved nut will taste. If black walnuts are new to you, take it from a confirmed walnut "nut": It's a winner!   ☻   Serves 8

1½ cups reduced-fat biscuit baking mix
¾ cup SPLENDA Granular
1 teaspoon baking powder
¾ cup fat-free milk
2 tablespoons vegetable oil
1 egg, or equivalent in egg substitute
1 teaspoon vanilla extract
¼ cup chopped black walnuts

Preheat oven to 350 degrees. Spray a 9-inch round cake pan with butter-flavored cooking spray. In a large bowl, combine baking mix, Splenda, and baking powder. Add milk, vegetable oil, egg, and vanilla extract. Mix gently just to combine using a sturdy spoon. Fold in black walnuts. Evenly spread batter into prepared cake pan. Bake for 22 to 26 minutes, or until a toothpick inserted in center comes out clean. Place pan on a wire rack and allow to cool completely. Cut into 8 servings.

HINT: If desired, frost with Grandma JO's Chocolate Glaze.

Each serving equals:

HE: 1 Bread • 1 Fat • ¼ Protein • 17 Optional Calories

168 Calories • 8 gm Fat • 4 gm Protein • 20 gm Carbohydrate • 329 mg Sodium • 87 mg Calcium • 1 gm Fiber

DIABETIC EXCHANGES: 1 Starch • 1 Fat

Pineapple Chocolate Chip Cake

For all you "pineapple people" out there, here's a party cake that blends chocolate, cinnamon, and nuts with that gold-medal fruit! Keep lots of pineapple on hand if you've got the shelf space—it adds sparkle to so many Healthy Exchanges dishes.

○ Serves 12

⅓ cup reduced-calorie margarine
1 cup SPLENDA Granular
2 eggs, or equivalent in egg substitute
2 (8-ounce) cans crushed pineapple, packed in fruit juice,
    drained, and ½ cup liquid reserved
¼ cup fat-free half & half
2¼ cups all-purpose flour
1½ teaspoons baking soda
½ teaspoon ground cinnamon
½ cup mini chocolate chips
¼ cup chopped pecans

Preheat oven to 350 degrees. Spray a Bundt pan with butter-flavored cooking spray. In a large bowl, combine margarine, Splenda, and eggs using a wire whisk. Stir in pineapple, reserved pineapple liquid, and half & half. In a small bowl, combine flour, baking soda, and cinnamon. Add flour mixture to margarine mixture. Mix gently just to combine using a sturdy spoon. Fold in chocolate chips and pecans. Evenly spread batter into prepared pan. Bake for 40 to 45 minutes, or until a toothpick inserted in center comes out clean. Place pan on a wire rack and let set for 15 minutes. Gently loosen cake from pan with a knife and invert onto a serving plate. Let set for at least 30 minutes. Cut into 12 servings.

Each serving equals:

HE: 1 Bread • 1 Fat • ⅓ Fruit • ½ Slider • 5 Optional Calories

199 Calories • 7 gm Fat • 4 gm Protein • 30 gm Carbohydrate • 237 mg Sodium • 23 mg Calcium • 2 gm Fiber

DIABETIC EXCHANGES: 1½ Starch/Carbohydrate • 1 Fat • ½ Fruit

Charming Cookies and Bars

Did you ever wonder who made the first cookies? *The Oxford History of Food* says that it was probably a Roman who mixed up a paste of wheat flour, fried it, and served it with honey. Later versions of cookies added sugar and eggs—and, by the 1700s, shortening. They only began coating cookies with chocolate in the years after World War II. And the word *cookie* actually comes from the Dutch word *koekje*, which means "little cake."

Okay, enough research and history—let's eat! I've got a terrific selection of cookies and bars sweetened with Splenda, and I hope you're planning to eat your way from one end of this chapter to the end. For you brownie lovers, head for the *Pecan Cocoa Brownies*, *Cheyanne's Fudgy Brownies* or *Cheesecake Topped Fudge Brownies*— yum! Still hungry? Good. Stir up *Josh's Walnut Triple Chocolate Bars*, *Chocolate Cappuccino Chip Bars*, *Apple Pie Cheesecake Bars*, or *Lemon Crumb Bars*. And for all you cookie fans, start with *Cranberry Walnut Oatmeal Cookies* and *Peanut Butter Cup Cookies*. Scrumptious!

Cookies and Bars Baking Tips

Even if you've been baking cookies for years, I bet I've got a few secrets that will help you make the best cookies you and your family have ever eaten!

1. For best results, you will need an extra-large bowl and a good-quality wire whisk. Here's why: I discovered that because the fat is greatly reduced in my recipes, you can

produce a crisper cookie by combining the margarine (and applesauce, if listed) with the Splenda in a very large bowl using a wire whisk. This allows extra air into the batter and makes for a better cookie. I also found out that if I used the largest mixing bowl I had (a huge metal bowl), I had more "room" to mix, which in turn made the cookies turn out better. So if you don't already have an extra-large mixing bowl and a good-quality wire whisk, now is the time to invest in both. When you start getting compliments every time you stir up another batch of cookies or bars, you'll be very glad you did!

2. Never over-stir the batter after the dry ingredients have been added, as this causes the cookies to turn out tough. Mix just enough to combine, *and no more*!

3. Try to have all your refrigerated ingredients at room temperature before starting to stir up a batch of cookies. It really makes a difference!

4. Some of my recipes will call for spraying the baking sheet with butter-flavored cooking spray; others will ask for an ungreased baking sheet. This is based on the amount of shortening in the recipe. Some people find that they have better luck baking cookies if they line their baking sheets with parchment paper or waxed paper. It does make for easier cleanup! This is a personal choice, so do whatever works best for you.

5. To ensure nicely rounded drop cookies, spoon the dough up using one spoon, and drop the dough onto the baking sheet with another spoon. *Don't use measuring spoons!* Use the tablespoons or teaspoons from your flatware set.

6. Try to make all cookies in a batch the same size, to ensure uniform baking. You'll also make certain that the nutrient info is as accurate as possible.

7. If you're baking one sheet of cookies at a time, bake them in the center of the oven. If you're baking two sheets,

arrange the oven racks so that the oven is divided into thirds (leaving an even distance between the racks).

8. Check cookies at the suggested minimum baking time. Try not to overbake. Using a metal spatula, immediately remove the cookies from the baking sheets to wire racks, because cookies continue to bake until they're removed from the hot-from-the-oven baking sheet.

9. Invest in enough cookie sheets so you can have more than one cooled baking sheet ready to put into the oven. Otherwise, if you try to use a baking sheet that is still warm (or worse, hot), the cookie dough will spread before it ever gets in the oven.

10. Drop cookies are done when the dough looks set and both the edges and bottoms of the cookies are lightly browned. Brownies and bars are done when either a cake tester or a toothpick inserted near the center comes out clean.

11. For best results, use only light-colored, shiny baking sheets with either no rim or a very low rim. Dark or discolored pans cause the cookies to burn on the bottom. Baking sheets that are too large may prevent proper heat circulation, which is necessary for even baking.

12. Store crisp, thin cookies in a container with a loose cover. Store soft cookies in a container with a tight-fitting cover. This will help keep the crisp cookies crisp and the soft cookies soft. Whichever kind of cookie you are storing, don't put it in a container until after it has completely cooled.

Cheyanne's Chocolate Chip Cookies

Ever since she was just a "mini" herself, my granddaughter Cheyanne has begged to stir in the mini chocolate chips when I was baking cookies. She does a great job, too, and she's patient enough to wait until the cookies have cooled before asking for her "pay"!

❂ Serves 12 (2 each)

> 6 tablespoons reduced-calorie margarine
> ¾ cup SPLENDA Granular
> 1 egg, or equivalent in egg substitute
> 1 teaspoon vanilla extract
> 1½ cups all-purpose flour
> ½ teaspoon baking soda
> ¼ teaspoon table salt
> ¾ cup mini chocolate chips

Preheat oven to 350 degrees. Spray 2 baking sheets with butter-flavored cooking spray. In a large bowl, combine margarine, Splenda, and egg using a wire whisk. Stir in vanilla extract. In a small bowl, combine flour, baking soda, and salt. Add flour mixture to margarine mixture. Mix gently just to combine using a sturdy spoon. Fold in chocolate chips. Drop batter by large tablespoonful onto prepared baking sheets to form 24 cookies. Lightly flatten cookies with the bottom of a glass sprayed with butter-flavored cooking spray. Bake for 6 to 8 minutes, or until lightly browned. Place baking sheets on wire racks and let set for 2 minutes. Remove cookies from baking sheets and continue to cool on wire racks.

Each serving equals:

HE: ¾ Fat • ⅔ Bread • ¾ Slider • 4 Optional Calories

146 Calories • 6 gm Fat • 3 gm Protein • 20 gm Carbohydrate • 176 mg Sodium • 9 mg Calcium • 1 gm Fiber

DIABETIC EXCHANGES: 1 Fat • 1 Starch/Carbohydrate

Peanut-Butter-Cup Cookies

Are peanut-butter cups on your Top Ten List of favorite candies? Join the club (and we've got lots of members!). These cookies honor one of the best pairings since love and marriage.

Serves 12 (2 each)

⅓ cup reduced-calorie margarine
¼ cup reduced-fat peanut butter
¾ cup SPLENDA Granular
2 eggs, or equivalent in egg substitute
1 teaspoon vanilla extract
1¼ cups all-purpose flour
½ teaspoon baking soda
¼ teaspoon table salt
12 sugar-free miniature peanut-butter cups, cut into small
  pieces

Preheat oven to 350 degrees. Spray 2 baking sheets with butter-flavored cooking spray. In a large bowl, combine margarine, peanut butter, Splenda, and eggs using a wire whisk. Stir in vanilla extract. In a small bowl, combine flour, baking soda, and salt. Add flour mixture to margarine mixture. Mix gently just to combine using a sturdy spoon. Fold in peanut-butter-cup pieces. Drop batter by tablespoonful onto prepared baking sheets to form 24 cookies. Lightly flatten cookies with the bottom of a glass sprayed with butter-flavored cooking spray. Bake for 7 to 9 minutes, or until lightly browned. Place baking sheets on wire racks and let set for 2 minutes. Remove cookies from baking sheets and continue to cool on wire racks.

Each serving equals:

HE: 1 Fat • ½ Bread • ½ Protein • ½ Slider • 11 Optional Calories

169 Calories • 9 gm Fat • 4 gm Protein • 18 gm Carbohydrate • 238 mg Sodium • 27 mg Calcium • 1 gm Fiber

DIABETIC EXCHANGES: 1½ Fat • 1½ Starch/Carbohydrate

Ranger Cookies

My grandsons are members of the Royal Rangers at church, and these cookies were designed for boys with very healthy appetites! They're fiber-rich and sweet, with lots of crunch.

● Serves 12 (2 each)

> ½ cup reduced-calorie margarine
> 1 cup SPLENDA Granular
> 1 egg, or equivalent in egg substitute
> 2 tablespoons fat-free milk
> 1 teaspoon vanilla extract
> 1 cup all-purpose flour
> 1 cup quick oats
> ½ teaspoon baking powder
> ½ teaspoon baking soda
> 1 cup cornflakes
> ¼ cup chopped dry-roasted peanuts

Preheat oven to 350 degrees. Spray 2 baking sheets with butter-flavored cooking spray. In a large bowl, combine margarine, Splenda, and egg using a wire whisk. Stir in milk and vanilla extract. In a small bowl, combine flour, oats, baking powder, and baking soda. Add flour mixture to margarine mixture. Mix gently just to combine using a sturdy spoon. Fold in cornflakes and peanuts. Shape dough into 24 (1-inch) balls. Place balls on prepared baking sheets. Lightly flatten cookies with the bottom of a glass sprayed with butter-flavored cooking spray. Bake for 8 to 12 minutes, or until lightly browned. Place baking sheets on wire racks and let set for 1 minute. Remove cookies from baking sheets and continue to cool on wire racks.

Each serving equals:

HE: 1 Bread • 1 Fat • 19 Optional Calories

134 Calories • 6 gm Fat • 3 gm Protein • 17 gm Carbohydrate • 189 mg Sodium • 23 mg Calcium • 1 gm Fiber

DIABETIC EXCHANGES: 1 Starch • 1 Fat

Chocolate Walnut Meringues

If you've never tried putting parchment on your baking sheets, you'll be delighted to see how they help you get these pretty little treats off in one piece! These are delicate and beautiful—and they melt in your mouth. ❂ Serves 12 (3 each)

6 egg whites
1 cup SPLENDA Granular
¼ teaspoon table salt
⅓ cup unsweetened cocoa powder
½ cup finely chopped walnuts

Preheat oven to 350 degrees. Line 3 baking sheets with parchment paper. In a large bowl, beat egg whites with an electric mixer on HIGH until soft peaks form. Add Splenda and salt. Continue beating on HIGH until stiff peaks form. Fold in cocoa powder and walnuts using a rubber spatula. Spoon 1-inch mounds about 1 inch apart on prepared baking sheets. Bake for 14 to 18 minutes, or until mounds are dry to the touch. Place baking sheets on wire racks and allow to cool completely. Store in airtight container.

HINT: Egg whites beat best at room temperature.

Each serving equals:

HE: ⅓ Protein • ⅓ Fat • 13 Optional Calories

55 Calories • 3 gm Fat • 3 gm Protein • 4 gm Carbohydrate • 77 mg Sodium • 9 mg Calcium • 1 gm Fiber

DIABETIC EXCHANGES: ½ Meat • ½ Fat

S'More Cookies

Camp memories grow sweeter as time passes, but why wait till there's a campfire and ants before you enjoy this classic outdoor treat? Gather the ingredients, sing a few camp songs, and invite your friends to munch on a few of these!

❍ Serves 12 (2 each)

½ cup reduced-calorie margarine
1 recipe Grandma JO's Sweetened Condensed Milk
½ cup SPLENDA Granular
2¼ cups graham-cracker crumbs
½ cup mini chocolate chips
1 cup miniature marshmallows

Preheat oven to 350 degrees. Spray 2 baking sheets with butter-flavored cooking spray. In a large bowl, combine margarine, Grandma JO's Sweetened Condensed Milk, and Splenda using a wire whisk. Add graham-cracker crumbs. Mix gently just to combine using a sturdy spoon. Fold in chocolate chips and marshmallows. Drop by tablespoonful onto prepared baking sheets to form 24 cookies. Lightly flatten cookies with the bottom of a glass sprayed with butter-flavored cooking spray. Bake for 10 to 14 minutes, or until lightly browned. Place baking sheets on wire racks and let set for 2 minutes. Remove cookies from baking sheets and continue to cool on wire racks.

HINT: Recipe for Grandma JO's Sweetened Condensed Milk appears in the last chapter.

Each serving equals:

HE: 1 Bread • 1 Fat • ¼ Fat-Free Milk • ½ Slider • 15 Optional Calories

183 Calories • 7 gm Fat • 4 gm Protein • 26 gm Carbohydrate • 232 mg Sodium • 108 mg Calcium • 1 gm Fiber

DIABETIC EXCHANGES: 1½ Starch/Other Carbohydrate • 1 Fat

Oatmeal Delite Cookies

Are you one of those kids whose mom spooned applesauce onto your oatmeal when you were little? Then you already know what a dynamite combination those two can be! Add some little surprises to every bite, and you'll be oh-so-pleased with the result. Phyllis, one of my recipe testers, supplied the name for this "delight."

◉ Serves 12 (2 each)

> ⅓ cup reduced-calorie margarine
> ½ cup SPLENDA Granular
> 2 eggs, or equivalent in egg substitute
> 1 cup unsweetened applesauce
> 1 cup + 2 tablespoons all-purpose flour
> 1 teaspoon baking powder
> 1½ cups quick oats
> 1 teaspoon apple-pie spice
> ½ cup seedless raisins
> ¼ cup mini chocolate chips
> ¼ cup chopped walnuts

Preheat oven to 375 degrees. Spray 2 baking sheets with butter-flavored cooking spray. In a large bowl, combine margarine, Splenda, and eggs using a wire whisk. Stir in applesauce. In a small bowl, combine flour, baking powder, oats, and apple-pie spice. Add flour mixture to margarine mixture. Mix gently just to combine using a sturdy spoon. Fold in raisins, chocolate chips, and walnuts. Drop batter by tablespoonful onto prepared baking sheets to form 24 cookies. Flatten each cookie with the tines of a fork. Bake for 10 to 12 minutes, or until lightly browned. Place cookies on wire racks and allow to cool completely.

Each serving equals:

HE: 1 Bread • 1 Fat • ½ Fruit • ¼ Protein • 16 Optional Calories

138 Calories • 6 gm Fat • 3 gm Protein • 18 gm Carbohydrate • 107 mg Sodium • 39 mg Calcium • 2 gm Fiber

DIABETIC EXCHANGES: 1 Starch • 1 Fat • ½ Fruit

Cranberry Walnut Oatmeal Cookies

If you've felt a bit stuck in the old oatmeal-raisin rut, here's a festive suggestion for something that will make your kids sit up and take notice: a blend of crunchy nuts and sweet red cranberries dried to even sweeter gems.   ☻   Serves 12 (2 each)

6 tablespoons + 2 teaspoons reduced-calorie margarine
¾ cup SPLENDA Granular
1 egg, or equivalent in egg substitute
1 teaspoon vanilla extract
½ cup all-purpose flour
1 cup quick oats
½ teaspoon baking soda
¼ teaspoon salt
½ cup craisins
¼ cup chopped walnuts

Preheat oven to 350 degrees. Spray 2 baking sheets with butter-flavored cooking spray. In a large bowl, combine margarine, Splenda, and egg using a wire whisk. Stir in vanilla extract. In a small bowl, combine flour, oats, baking soda, and salt. Add flour mixture to margarine mixture. Mix gently just to combine using a sturdy spoon. Fold in craisins and walnuts. Drop by tablespoonful onto prepared baking sheets to form 24 cookies. Lightly flatten cookies with the bottom of a glass sprayed with butter-flavored cooking spray. Bake for 7 to 9 minutes, or until lightly browned. Place baking sheets on wire racks and let set for 2 minutes. Remove cookies from baking sheets and continue to cool on wire racks.

Each serving equals:

HE: 1 Fat • ½ Bread • ⅓ Fruit • 19 Optional Calories

113 Calories • 5 gm Fat • 2 gm Protein • 15 gm Carbohydrate • 183 mg Sodium • 10 mg Calcium • 1 gm Fiber

DIABETIC EXCHANGES: 1 Fat • 1 Starch/Carbohydrate

Chocolate Chip Brownies

There are some brownie purists who want to taste only brownie in each bite, but I'm of the school that appreciates "add-ins"! Walnuts and chocolate chips add very few additional calories, but they contribute so much to the pleasure that comes with each mouthful!

● Serves 12 (2 each)

> ½ cup reduced-calorie margarine
> 1 cup SPLENDA Granular
> 3 eggs, or equivalent in egg substitute
> 1 tablespoon fat-free milk
> 2 teaspoons vanilla extract
> 1¼ cups all-purpose flour
> ¼ cup unsweetened cocoa powder
> ¼ teaspoon baking soda
> ¾ cup mini chocolate chips
> ¼ cup chopped walnuts

Preheat oven to 350 degrees. Spray a 7-by-11-inch biscuit pan with butter-flavored cooking spray. In a large bowl, combine margarine, Splenda, eggs, and milk using a wire whisk. Stir in vanilla extract. In a small bowl, combine flour, cocoa powder, and baking soda. Add flour mixture to margarine mixture. Mix gently just to combine using a sturdy spoon. Fold in chocolate chips and walnuts. Evenly spread batter into prepared pan. Bake for 15 to 20 minutes, or until a toothpick inserted in center comes out clean. Place pan on a wire rack and allow to cool completely. Cut into 24 bars.

Each serving equals:

HE: 1 Fat • ¾ Bread • ¼ Protein • ¾ Slider • 10 Optional Calories

186 Calories • 10 gm Fat • 4 gm Protein • 20 gm Carbohydrate • 137 mg Sodium • 20 mg Calcium • 2 gm Fiber

DIABETIC EXCHANGES: 1½ Fat • 1½ Starch/Carbohydrate

Cheyanne's Fudgy Brownies

What makes a brownie extra-fudgy? Well, stirring in lots of grand-kid love is a great start, but this recipe has a deeper chocolate taste for several good reasons—some extra cocoa powder (use the best cocoa powder you can afford!), some applesauce, and a bit more egg. ☻ Serves 12 (2 each)

> 6 tablespoons + 2 teaspoons reduced-calorie margarine
> 2 cups SPLENDA Granular
> 4 eggs, or equivalent in egg substitute
> ¾ cup unsweetened applesauce
> 1 tablespoon vanilla extract
> 1 cup cake flour
> ¾ cup unsweetened cocoa powder
> 1 teaspoon baking powder
> ¼ teaspoon table salt
> ¼ cup chopped walnuts

Preheat oven to 350 degrees. Spray a 7-by-11-inch biscuit pan with butter-flavored cooking spray. In a large bowl, combine margarine, Splenda, and eggs using a wire whisk. Stir in applesauce and vanilla extract. In a small bowl, combine flour, cocoa powder, baking powder, and salt. Add flour mixture to margarine mixture. Mix gently just to combine using a sturdy spoon. Fold in walnuts. Spread batter evenly into prepared pan. Bake for 20 to 26 minutes, or until a toothpick inserted in center comes out clean.. Place pan on a wire rack and allow to cool completely. Cut into 24 bars.

Each serving equals:

HE: 1 Fat • ½ Bread • ¼ Protein • ¼ Slider • 10 Optional Calories

143 Calories • 7 gm Fat • 4 gm Protein • 16 gm Carbohydrate • 182 mg Sodium • 41 mg Calcium • 2 gm Fiber

DIABETIC EXCHANGES: 1 Fat • 1 Starch/Carbohydrate

Coconut Raspberry Cheesecake Brownies

I can think of some commercial brownie makers who'd be proud to put these on the bakery shelf, but you can stir them up at home and win all the applause yourself! I tried this with other spreadable fruits and chose raspberry as my favorite, but if you love apricot or peach, give it a try. ☻ Serves 12 (2 each)

1 (8-ounce) package fat-free cream cheese
3 eggs, or equivalent in egg substitute ☆
1 cup SPLENDA Granular ☆
¾ cup raspberry spreadable fruit
2 tablespoons fat-free sour cream
½ cup fat-free half & half
1 teaspoon coconut extract
¾ cup reduced-fat biscuit baking mix
¼ cup unsweetened cocoa powder
¼ cup chopped walnuts
¼ cup mini chocolate chips
2 tablespoons flaked coconut

Preheat oven to 375 degrees. Spray a 7-by-11-inch biscuit pan with butter-flavored cooking spray. In a medium bowl, stir cream cheese with a sturdy spoon until softened. Add 2 eggs, ¼ cup Splenda, and spreadable fruit. Mix well to combine. Set aside. In a large bowl, combine sour cream, half & half, coconut extract, and remaining 1 egg. Stir in remaining ¾ cup Splenda. Add baking mix and cocoa powder. Mix gently just to combine. Evenly spread batter into prepared pan. Drop cream cheese mixture by tablespoonful over batter. Carefully spread cream cheese mixture to cover batter, using a rubber spatula. In a small bowl, combine walnuts, chocolate chips, and coconut. Sprinkle mixture evenly over top. Bake for 18 to 22 minutes, or until a toothpick inserted in center comes out clean. Place pan on a wire rack and allow to cool completely. Cut into 24 bars.

Each serving equals:

HE: ⅔ Protein • ½ Fruit • ⅓ Bread • ½ Slider • 2 Optional Calories

165 Calories • 5 gm Fat • 6 gm Protein • 24 gm Carbohydrate • 218 mg Sodium • 86 mg Calcium • 1 gm Fiber

DIABETIC EXCHANGES: 1 Starch/Carbohydrate • ½ Meat • ½ Fruit • ½ Fat

Cheesecake Topped Fudge Brownies

I've seen Internet ads for specialty brownies topped with all sorts of goodies, but their prices can be very high, especially when you figure in the cost of shipping. Instead, try making these recklessly rich brownies in your own kitchen—and putting the money you save toward a new baking pan or a pair of pretty shoes!

○ Serves 12

½ cup reduced-calorie margarine ☆
¼ cup fat-free sour cream
3 eggs, or equivalent in egg substitute ☆
1 tablespoon vanilla extract ☆
1 cup SPLENDA Granular
¼ cup unsweetened cocoa powder
¾ cup cake flour
1 (8-ounce) package fat-free cream cheese
1 tablespoon cornstarch
1 recipe Grandma JO's Sweetened Condensed Milk
½ cup mini chocolate chips

Preheat oven to 350 degrees. Spray a 7-by-11-inch biscuit pan with butter-flavored cooking spray. In a large bowl, combine 6 tablespoons margarine, sour cream, 2 eggs, and 1 teaspoon vanilla extract using a wire whisk. Add Splenda, cocoa powder, and flour. Mix gently just to combine using a sturdy spoon. Evenly spread batter into prepared pan. In another large bowl, stir cream cheese with a sturdy spoon until softened. Stir in remaining 2 tablespoons margarine and cornstarch. Add Grandma JO's Sweetened Condensed Milk, remaining 1 egg, and remaining 2 teaspoons vanilla extract. Mix gently just to combine using a sturdy spoon. Stir in chocolate chips. Carefully spread mixture over brownie mixture. Bake for 33 to 37 minutes, or until a toothpick inserted in center comes out clean. Place pan on a wire rack and allow to cool completely. Cut into 12 bars.

1. Recipe for Grandma JO's Sweetened Condensed Milk appears in the last chapter.
2. Good frosted with Grandma JO's Chocolate Glaze.

Each serving equals:

HE: 1 Fat • ½ Protein • ⅓ Fat-Free Milk • ⅓ Bread • ½ Slider • 19 Optional Calories

179 Calories • 7 gm Fat • 8 gm Protein • 21 gm Carbohydrate • 252 mg Sodium • 175 mg Calcium • 1 gm Fiber

DIABETIC EXCHANGES: 1 Fat • 1 Other Carbohydrate • ½ Meat

Banana Blondies

Is it true that blondes have more fun? (As a woman with golden locks, I like to think so!) Well, even brunettes and redheads can give being blonde a try with these utterly original blond brownies that are amazingly moist and rich.   ○   Serves 12 (2 each)

⅓ *cup reduced-calorie margarine*
1⅓ *cups SPLENDA Granular*
1 *egg, or equivalent in egg substitute*
⅓ *cup unsweetened applesauce*
⅔ *cup (2 medium) mashed ripe bananas*
1 *teaspoon vanilla extract*
1½ *cups reduced-fat biscuit baking mix*
2 *teaspoons baking powder*
¼ *teaspoon table salt*
½ *cup mini chocolate chips*
½ *cup chopped walnuts*

Preheat oven to 350 degrees. Spray a 7-by-11-inch biscuit pan with butter-flavored cooking spray. In a large bowl, combine margarine, Splenda, and egg using a wire whisk. Stir in applesauce, mashed bananas, and vanilla extract. In a small bowl, combine baking mix, baking powder, and salt. Add baking mix mixture to margarine mixture. Mix well to combine using a sturdy spoon. Fold in chocolate chips and walnuts. Evenly spread batter into prepared pan. Bake for 25 to 30 minutes, or until a toothpick inserted in center comes out clean. Place pan on a wire rack and allow to cool completely. Cut into 24 bars.

Each serving equals:

HE: 1 Fat • ⅔ Bread • ⅓ Fruit • ¼ Protein • ½ Slider • 8 Optional Calories

181 Calories • 9 gm Fat • 3 gm Protein • 22 gm Carbohydrate • 356 mg Sodium • 66 mg Calcium • 1 gm Fiber

DIABETIC EXCHANGES: 1½ Starch/Carbohydrate, 1 Fat

Raspberry Chocolate Chip Bars

I'm a big fan of bar cookies because they bake up so easily in just one pan. These fruit-topped chocolate-chippers are irresistible, so you might want to bake more than a dozen!

● Serves 12 (2 each)

> ⅓ cup reduced-calorie margarine
> ¾ cup Splenda Granular
> ¾ cup all-purpose flour
> 1 cup quick oats
> ½ teaspoon baking soda
> ½ teaspoon table salt
> ¾ cup raspberry spreadable fruit
> ½ cup mini chocolate chips

Preheat oven to 375 degrees. Spray a 7-by-11-inch biscuit pan with butter-flavored cooking spray. In a large bowl, combine margarine and Splenda using a wire whisk. In a small bowl, combine flour, oats, baking soda, and salt. Add flour mixture to margarine mixture. Mix gently to combine using a sturdy spoon. Reserve ½ cup of the mixture. Pat remaining mixture in bottom of prepared pan. Carefully spread spreadable fruit over crumb crust. In a small bowl, combine reserved mixture and chocolate chips. Evenly sprinkle mixture over top. Bake for 25 to 30 minutes, or until a toothpick inserted in center comes out clean. Place pan on a wire rack and allow to cool completely. Cut into 24 bars.

Each serving equals:

HE: ⅔ Bread • ⅔ Fruit • ⅔ Fat • ½ Slider • 1 Optional Calorie

157 Calories • 5 gm Fat • 2 gm Protein • 26 gm Carbohydrate • 210 mg Sodium • 8 mg Calcium • 1 gm Fiber

DIABETIC EXCHANGES: 1½ Starch/Carbohydrate • 1 Fat

Chocolate Nut Bars

If you've never cooked with sweetened condensed milk, you may not know how it can transform a recipe for favorite sweets! These fudgy, nutty delights win lots of votes from every kid who's ever tried them, and they're just great for bake sales, too.

☻ Serves 12 (2 each)

1½ cups graham-cracker crumbs
⅓ cup reduced-calorie margarine
1 recipe Grandma JO's Sweetened Condensed Milk
¼ cup hot water
¼ cup unsweetened cocoa powder
½ cup SPLENDA Granular
2 teaspoons vanilla extract
6 tablespoons mini chocolate chips
½ cup chopped walnuts

Preheat oven to 375 degrees. Spray a 7-by-11-inch biscuit pan with butter-flavored cooking spray. In a medium bowl, combine graham-cracker crumbs and margarine. Mix well using a pastry blender or 2 forks until mixture becomes crumbly. Pat mixture into prepared pan. Bake for 8 minutes. Place pan on a wire rack. Lower oven temperature to 350 degrees. In a medium saucepan, combine Grandma JO's Sweetened Condensed Milk, hot water, cocoa powder, Splenda, and vanilla extract. Cook over medium heat until mixture is smooth and just starts to boil, stirring constantly using a wire whisk. Spread mixture evenly over crust using a rubber spatula. Evenly sprinkle chocolate chips and walnuts over top. Continue baking for 25 to 30 minutes, or until a toothpick inserted in center comes out clean. Place pan on a wire rack and allow to cool completely. Cut into 24 bars.

HINT: Recipe for Grandma JO's Sweetened Condensed Milk appears in the last chapter.

Each serving equals:

HE: 1 Fat • ⅔ Bread • ⅓ Fat-Free Milk • ¼ Slider • 10 Optional Calories

160 Calories • 8 gm Fat • 5 gm Protein • 17 gm Carbohydrate • 166 mg Sodium • 113 mg Calcium • 2 gm Fiber

DIABETIC EXCHANGES: 1½ Starch/Carbohydrate • 1 Fat

Chocolate Cherry Bars

Imagine the splendid glory of a perfect chocolate covered cherry—and now, imagine that flavor in a beautiful bar cookie. Is your mouth watering in anticipation yet? Mm-mm . . .

● Serves 12 (2 each)

>   6 tablespoons reduced-calorie margarine
>   1 cup SPLENDA Granular
>   ¼ cup fat-free sour cream
>   2 tablespoons Land O Lakes fat-free half & half
>   4 eggs, or equivalent in egg substitute ☆
>   1 teaspoon almond extract
>   ½ cup unsweetened cocoa powder
>   1¼ cups reduced-fat biscuit baking mix ☆
>   1 recipe Grandma JO's Sweetened Condensed Milk
>   ¼ cup mini chocolate chips
>   12 maraschino cherries, chopped and drained

Preheat oven to 350 degrees. Spray a 7-by-11-inch biscuit pan with butter-flavored cooking spray. In a large bowl, combine margarine and Splenda using a wire whisk. Stir in sour cream, half & half, 3 eggs, and ½ teaspoon almond extract. Add cocoa powder and ¾ cup baking mix. Mix well to combine using a sturdy spoon. Spread batter evenly into prepared pan. Bake for 10 minutes. Meanwhile, in a medium bowl, combine remaining egg and Grandma JO's Sweetened Condensed Milk. Stir in remaining ½ teaspoon almond extract. Add remaining ½ cup baking mix. Mix well to combine using a wire whisk. Carefully spread mixture over partially baked layer. Evenly sprinkle chocolate chips and chopped maraschino cherries over top. Continue baking for 18 to 22 minutes or until filling is set. Place pan on a wire rack and allow to cool completely. Cut into 24 bars.

HINT: Recipe for Grandma JO's Sweetened Condensed Milk appears in the last chapter.

Each serving equals:

HE: ¾ Fat • ½ Bread • ⅓ Fat-Free Milk • ¼ Protein • ½ Slider • 10 Optional Calories

166 Calories • 6 gm Fat • 5 gm Protein • 23 gm Carbohydrate • 275 mg Sodium • 130 mg Calcium • 1 gm Fiber

DIABETIC EXCHANGES: 1½ Starch/Carbohydrate • 1 Fat

Josh's Walnut Triple Chocolate Bars

My grandson Josh likes to watch me measure out the chocolate syrup, enjoying the "plop, plop" sound it makes as I pour it into the measuring cup. Walnuts are his nut of choice, so I named these for him. ❂ Serves 12 (2 each)

1 cup + 2 tablespoons graham-cracker crumbs
¼ cup unsweetened cocoa powder
½ cup SPLENDA Granular ☆
⅓ cup + 1 tablespoon reduced-calorie margarine
1 recipe Grandma JO's Sweetened Condensed Milk
¼ cup reduced-calorie chocolate syrup
2 eggs, or equivalent in egg substitute ☆
1 teaspoon vanilla extract
3 tablespoons all-purpose flour
¼ cup chopped walnuts
⅓ cup mini chocolate chips

Preheat oven to 350 degrees. Spray a 7-by-11-inch biscuit pan with butter-flavored cooking spray. In a large bowl, combine graham-cracker crumbs, cocoa powder, and ¼ cup Splenda. Add margarine. Mix well using a pastry blender or 2 forks until mixture becomes crumbly. Press mixture firmly in bottom of prepared pan. In same large bowl, combine Grandma JO's Sweetened Condensed Milk, chocolate syrup, 1 egg, and vanilla extract. Mix well using a wire whisk. Blend in flour. Fold in walnuts. Evenly spread mixture over prepared crust. Sprinkle chocolate chips evenly over top. Bake for 22 to 26 minutes, or until filling is set. Place pan on a wire rack and allow to cool completely. Cut into 24 bars.

HINT: Recipe for Grandma JO's Sweetened Condensed Milk appears in the last chapter.

Each serving equals:

HE: 1 Fat • ½ Bread • ⅓ Fat-Free Milk • ¼ Protein • ½ Slider • 2 Optional Calories

164 Calories • 8 gm Fat • 5 gm Protein • 18 gm Carbohydrate • 174 mg Sodium • 115 mg Calcium • 1 gm Fiber

DIABETIC EXCHANGES: 1½ Starch/Carbohydrate • 1 Fat

Chocolate Cappuccino Chip Bars

Once it was a sophisticated Italian coffee drink that was served only in Italian cafés, but these days, you can find cappuccino in everything from milk shakes to doughnuts. I'm a big fan of chocolate and coffee, spiced with cinnamon, so I stirred some into a classic bar cookie recipe. Yum, yum!

Serves 16 (2 each)

½ cup reduced-calorie margarine
½ cup unsweetened applesauce
1½ cups SPLENDA Granular
2 eggs, or equivalent in egg substitute
¼ cup fat-free half & half
1 teaspoon vanilla extract
1¾ cups all-purpose flour
⅓ cup unsweetened cocoa powder
1 tablespoon ground cinnamon
2 teaspoons instant coffee crystals
1 teaspoon baking powder
1 teaspoon baking soda
¼ teaspoon table salt
¾ cup mini chocolate chips

Preheat oven to 350 degrees. Spray a 9-by-13-inch cake pan with butter-flavored cooking spray. In a large bowl, combine margarine, applesauce, and Splenda using a wire whisk. Stir in eggs, half & half, and vanilla extract. In a small bowl, combine flour, cocoa powder, cinnamon, coffee crystals, baking powder, baking soda, and salt. Add flour mixture to margarine mixture. Mix gently just to combine using a sturdy spoon. Fold in chocolate chips. Evenly spread batter into prepared cake pan. Bake for 14 to 18 minutes, or until a toothpick inserted in center comes out clean. Place pan on a wire rack and allow to cool completely. Cut into 32 bars.

Each serving equals:

HE: **¾ Bread • ¾ Fat • ½ Slider • 3 Optional Calories**

146 Calories • 6 gm Fat • 3 gm Protein • 20 gm Carbohydrate • 218 mg Sodium • 31 mg Calcium • 2 gm Fiber

DIABETIC EXCHANGES: **1½ Starch • ½ Fat**

Lemon Crumb Bars

Bar cookies are great for lunchboxes and bags because they tend to be sturdier than other kinds of cookies—and they travel well. What a nice surprise it would be to find a couple of these waiting for you when lunch hour rolls around! ☻ Serves 12 (2 each)

> 1 cup + 2 tablespoons reduced-fat biscuit baking mix
> ¾ cup SPLENDA Granular
> 1 teaspoon baking powder
> ¼ cup reduced-calorie margarine
> 21 small fat-free saltine crackers made into fine crumbs
> 2 eggs, or equivalent in egg substitute ☆
> 1 recipe Grandma JO's Sweetened Condensed Milk
> ½ cup lemon juice

Preheat oven to 350 degrees. Spray a 7-by-11-inch biscuit pan with butter-flavored cooking spray. In a large bowl, combine baking mix, Splenda, and baking powder. Add margarine. Mix well using a pastry blender or 2 forks until mixture becomes crumbly. Stir in cracker crumbs. Reserve ¾ cup crumb mixture. Press remaining crumb mixture firmly in bottom of prepared pan. Bake for 5 minutes. Meanwhile, in a medium bowl, beat eggs with a wire whisk until frothy. Add Grandma JO's Sweetened Condensed Milk and lemon juice. Mix well to combine using a wire whisk. Carefully spread mixture over partially baked crust. Sprinkle reserved crumb mixture over top. Lightly spray top with butter-flavored cooking spray. Continue baking for 26 to 28 minutes, or until filling is set. Place pan on a wire rack and allow to cool completely. Cut into 24 bars.

HINT: Recipe for Grandma JO's Sweetened Condensed Milk appears in the last chapter.

Each serving equals:

HE: ¾ Bread • ½ Fat • ⅓ Fat-Free Milk • ¼ Slider • 1 Optional Calorie

127 Calories • 3 gm Fat • 5 gm Protein • 20 gm Carbohydrate • 326 mg Sodium • 136 mg Calcium • 1 gm Fiber

DIABETIC EXCHANGES: 1½ Starch/Carbohydrate • ½ Fat

Creamy Lime Coconut Bars

There's something so tropical about the flavor of lime, and the color also suggests warm climates and tangy taste treats. These would be perfect for serving to guests on the verandah of an island estate, but they're equally ideal for offering to guests on a sultry summer night in Iowa! ◑ Serves 8 (2 each)

> 1 recipe Grandma JO's Sweetened Condensed Milk
> ½ cup lime juice
> 1 tablespoon cornstarch
> 3 or 4 drops green food coloring
> ¾ cup all-purpose flour
> ½ cup SPLENDA Granular
> 2 tablespoons finely chopped pecans
> ¼ cup reduced-calorie margarine
> ¼ cup flaked coconut

Preheat oven to 350 degrees. Spray a 7-by-11-inch biscuit pan with butter-flavored cooking spray. In a large bowl, combine Grandma JO's Sweetened Condensed Milk, lime juice, cornstarch, and green food coloring. Set aside. In a medium bowl, combine flour, Splenda, and pecans. Add margarine. Mix well using a pastry blender or 2 forks until mixture becomes crumbly. Pat mixture evenly into prepared pan. Bake for 8 minutes. Evenly spread milk mixture over hot crust. Sprinkle coconut evenly over top. Continue baking for 9 to 11 minutes, or until filling is set. Place pan on a wire rack and allow to cool completely. Cut into 16 bars.

HINT: Recipe for Grandma JO's Sweetened Condensed Milk appears in the last chapter.

Each serving equals:

HE: 1 Fat • ½ Fat-Free Milk • ½ Bread • ¼ Slider • 7 Optional Calories

153 Calories • 5 gm Fat • 6 gm Protein • 21 gm Carbohydrate • 137 mg Sodium • 157 mg Calcium • 1 gm Fiber

DIABETIC EXCHANGES: 1 Fat • 1 Starch/Carbohydrate • ½ Fat-Free Milk

Coconut Apricot Bars

I wonder how many tiny apricots it takes to make a jar of spreadable fruit. I bet it's a LOT! That's why it's so delectably sweet and sunny, perfect for topping a cookie and putting a smile on everyone's faces. ❤ Serves 12 (2 each)

> 1 cup quick oats
> 1½ cups reduced-fat biscuit baking mix
> ¾ cup SPLENDA Granular
> ¼ cup flaked coconut ☆
> ½ cup reduced-calorie margarine
> 1 cup + 2 tablespoons apricot spreadable fruit

Preheat oven to 350 degrees. Spray a 9-by-13-inch cake pan with butter-flavored cooking spray. In a large bowl, combine oats, baking mix, Splenda, and 2 tablespoons coconut. Add margarine. Mix well using a pastry blender or 2 forks until mixture becomes crumbly. Pat ⅔ of mixture into prepared cake pan. In a small bowl, stir spreadable fruit until softened. Carefully spread spreadable fruit over crust. Evenly sprinkle remaining crumb mixture over fruit. Sprinkle remaining 2 tablespoons coconut over top. Bake for 18 to 22 minutes, or until filling is set. Place pan on a wire rack and allow to cool completely. Cut into 24 bars.

Each serving equals:

HE: 1 Bread • 1 Fruit • 1 Fat • 11 Optional Calories

190 Calories • 6 gm Fat • 2 gm Protein • 32 gm Carbohydrate • 269 mg Sodium • 20 mg Calcium • 1 gm Fiber

DIABETIC EXCHANGES: 1 Starch • 1 Fruit • 1 Fat

Banana Bars

I could tell you about how much potassium bananas have and how nutritious they are, but all you really need to know is that these taste GOOD to the very last crumb. Bananas keep their moistness, even in a hot oven.   ☻   Serves 8 (2 each)

> ⅓ cup reduced-calorie margarine
> 1 cup SPLENDA Granular
> 2 eggs, or equivalent in egg substitute
> 1 cup (3 medium) mashed ripe bananas
> 1 cup all-purpose flour
> 1 teaspoon baking powder
> ½ teaspoon baking soda
> ¼ teaspoon table salt
> ½ teaspoon ground cinnamon

Preheat oven to 350 degrees. Spray a 9-by-9-inch cake pan with butter-flavored cooking spray. In a large bowl, combine margarine, Splenda, and eggs using a wire whisk. Stir in bananas. In a small bowl, combine flour, baking powder, baking soda, salt, and cinnamon. Add flour mixture to margarine mixture. Mix gently just to combine using a sturdy spoon. Spread batter evenly into prepared pan. Bake for 25 to 30 minutes, or until a toothpick inserted in center comes out clean. Place pan on a wire rack and allow to cool completely. Cut into 16 bars.

HINT: If desired, lightly dust with Grandma JO's Powdered Sugar.

Each serving equals:

HE: 1 Fat • ¾ Fruit • ⅔ Bread • ¼ Protein • 12 Optional Calories

141 Calories • 5 gm Fat • 3 gm Protein • 21 gm Carbohydrate • 309 mg Sodium • 43 mg Calcium • 1 gm Fiber

DIABETIC EXCHANGES: 1 Fat • 1 Fruit • ½ Starch

Holiday Raisin Bars

Instead of making the same cookie you always do for the holiday cookie exchange, why not add a new recipe to your festive seasonal repertoire? Leave a couple of these for Santa, and you're bound to find happy surprises under your tree Christmas morning!

○ Serves 12 (2 each)

¼ cup reduced-calorie margarine
½ cup SPLENDA Granular
2 eggs, or equivalent in egg substitute
¼ cup fat-free half & half
2 tablespoons water
1½ teaspoons vanilla extract
¾ cup + 2 tablespoons all-purpose flour
¼ cup graham-cracker crumbs
1 teaspoon baking soda
⅛ teaspoon table salt
1 teaspoon ground cinnamon
1 cup seedless raisins

Preheat oven to 350 degrees. Spray a 7-by-11-inch biscuit pan with butter-flavored cooking spray. In a large bowl, combine margarine, Splenda, and eggs using a wire whisk. Stir in half & half, water, and vanilla extract. In a small bowl, combine flour, graham cracker crumbs, baking soda, salt, and cinnamon. Add flour mixture to margarine mixture. Mix gently just to combine using a sturdy spoon. Fold in raisins. Evenly spread batter into prepared pan. Bake for 15 to 20 minutes, or until a toothpick inserted in center comes out clean. Place pan on a wire rack and allow to cool completely. Cut into 24 bars.

Each serving equals:

HE: ⅔ Fruit • ½ Bread • ½ Fat • 14 Optional Calories

115 Calories • 3 gm Fat • 3 gm Protein • 19 gm Carbohydrate • 198 mg Sodium • 15 mg Calcium • 1 gm Fiber

DIABETIC EXCHANGES: 1 Fruit • ½ Starch • ½ Fat

Cherry Cheese Bars

Sometimes you just don't want to stir up an entire cherry cheese-cake, or maybe you'd like a version that's easy to pack and eat on the road. If you long for a taste of cherries hugged by rich and creamy goodness, these bars will satisfy your desire!

❍ Serves 12 (2 each)

1¼ cups all-purpose flour
1¼ cups SPLENDA Granular ☆
6 tablespoons + 2 teaspoons reduced-calorie margarine
¼ cup finely chopped walnuts
¼ cup flaked coconut
2 (8-ounce) packages fat-free cream cheese
2 eggs, or equivalent in egg substitute
1 teaspoon coconut extract
1 (20-ounce) can sugar-free cherry pie filling

Preheat oven to 350 degrees. Spray a 9-by-13-inch cake pan with butter-flavored cooking spray. In a large bowl, combine flour and ½ cup Splenda. Add margarine. Mix well using a pastry blender or 2 forks until mixture becomes crumbly. Stir in walnuts and coconut. Reserve ½ cup crumb mixture. Pat remaining mixture into prepared pan. Bake for 8 to 10 minutes, or until edges are lightly brown. Meanwhile, in a large bowl, stir cream cheese with a sturdy spoon until softened. Add eggs, remaining ¾ cup Splenda, and coconut extract. Mix well to combine using a wire whisk. Evenly spread cream cheese filling over hot crust. Continue baking for 15 minutes. Carefully spread cherry pie filling over partially baked cream cheese layer. Sprinkle remaining crumb mixture over cherry layer. Continue baking for 15 minutes. Place pan on a wire rack and allow to cool completely. Refrigerate for at least 2 hours. Cut into 24 bars.

HINT: If you can't find purchased sugar-free cherry pie filling, use Grandma JO's Fruit Pie Filling.

Each serving equals:

HE: 1 Protein • 1 Fat • ½ Bread • ⅓ Fruit • 17 Optional Calories

170 Calories • 6 gm Fat • 9 gm Protein • 20 gm Carbohydrate • 326 mg Sodium • 182 mg Calcium • 1 gm Fiber

DIABETIC EXCHANGES: 1 Starch/Other Carbohydrate • 1 Meat • 1 Fat

Apple Pie Cheesecake Bars

I think cheesecake all by itself is absolutely scrumptious, but I think it's fun to create new toppings for that culinary all-star. What could be more all-American—or impossible to resist—than good old apple-pie? You might just start singing "God Bless America"!

◐ Serves 12 (2 each)

> 1½ cups quick oats ☆
> ¾ cup reduced-fat biscuit baking mix
> 1¼ cups + 2 tablespoons SPLENDA Granular ☆
> ⅓ cup reduced-calorie margarine
> 2 (8-ounce) packages fat-free cream cheese
> 2 eggs, or equivalent in egg substitute
> 1 teaspoon vanilla extract
> 1 cup (1 medium) tart cooking apples, cored, peeled, and
>   finely chopped
> ½ cup seedless raisins
> 1 teaspoon apple-pie spice

Preheat oven to 350 degrees. Spray a 7-by-11-inch biscuit pan with butter-flavored cooking spray. In a large bowl, combine 1¼ cups oats, baking mix, and ¾ cup Splenda. Add margarine. Mix well using a pastry blender or 2 forks until mixture becomes crumbly. Reserve ½ cup of crumb mixture. Evenly pat remaining crumbs into prepared pan. Bake for 10 minutes. Meanwhile, in a large bowl, stir cream cheese with a sturdy spoon until softened. Add eggs, remaining ½ cup Splenda, and vanilla extract. Mix well to combine using a wire whisk. Stir in chopped apples and raisins. Spread cream cheese filling over crust. In a small bowl, combine reserved crumb mixture, remaining ¼ cup oats, remaining 2 tablespoons Splenda, and apple-pie spice. Evenly sprinkle crumb mixture over cream cheese mixture. Continue baking for 30 to 35 minutes. Place pan on a wire rack and allow to cool completely. Cut into 24 bars.

Each serving equals:

HE: 1 Bread • ¾ Protein • ⅔ Fat • ½ Fruit • ¼ Slider • 6 Optional Calories

164 Calories • 4 gm Fat • 9 gm Protein • 23 gm Carbohydrate • 389 mg Sodium • 195 mg Calcium • 2 gm Fiber

DIABETIC EXCHANGES: 1 Starch • ½ Meat • ½ Fruit • ½ Fat

Five Layer Bars

Join me in a little dessert "geology" as we layer sweet goodies, one on the top of the next! These bars are full of tasty discoveries that are unearthed with every bite you take.

❂ Serves 12 (2 each)

> ¼ cup reduced-calorie margarine
> ¼ cup fat-free sour cream
> 2 tablespoons SPLENDA Granular
> 1½ cups graham cracker crumbs
> 1 recipe Grandma JO's Sweetened Condensed Milk
> 1 teaspoon almond extract
> ½ cup flaked coconut
> ¼ cup chopped slivered almonds
> ½ cup mini chocolate chips

Preheat oven to 350 degrees. Spray a 7-by-11-inch biscuit pan with butter-flavored cooking spray. In a large bowl, combine margarine and sour cream using a wire whisk. Stir in Splenda and graham cracker crumbs. Pat mixture into prepared biscuit pan. In a small bowl, combine Grandma JO's Sweetened Condensed Milk and almond extract. Carefully spread mixture over crust using a rubber spatula. Sprinkle coconut, almonds, and chocolate chips evenly over top. Press down lightly with a spatula. Bake for 22 to 26 minutes, or until lightly browned. Place pan on a wire rack and allow to cool completely. Cut into 24 bars.

HINT: Recipe for Grandma JO's Sweetened Condensed Milk appears in the last chapter.

Each serving equals:

HE: ⅔ Bread • ⅔ Fat • ⅓ Fat-Free Milk • ¾ Slider • 3 Optional Calories

163 Calories • 7 gm Fat • 5 gm Protein • 20 gm Carbohydrate • 166 mg Sodium • 120 mg Calcium • 1 gm Fiber

DIABETIC EXCHANGES: 1½ Starch/Carbohydrate • 1 Fat

Delectable

Desserts

No matter how much anyone eats of the salad, the soup, and the main course, you'll find that everyone saves room for dessert! (I've heard one man tell his kids, "I've got a pocket inside my tummy just for that purpose!") Dessert is like the period in a sentence—what goes before it is just not complete until it's added. However delicious or satisfying the hearty courses that precede dessert, most diners want something sweet before departing from the table.

This chapter is where I've chosen to highlight some grand finales that don't fit into any of the other categories: luscious puddings like *Daddy's Bread Pudding, Southern Banana Pudding*, and *Lemon-Meringue Pudding Cups*; cozy cobblers and crisps, including *Apple Cinnamon Cobbler, Old-Time Apple Betty*, and *Grande Strawberry Rhubarb Crisp*; and some delights that are a little bit of several things: *Aaron's Hot Fudge Pudding Cake, Cherry Almond Cobbler Criss Cross, Candy Bar Shortcakes*, and *Raspberry Orange Crumble*.

Dessert-Baking Tips

For divine desserts, you'll want to keep these handy half dozen baking tips in mind—and don't be surprised if the applause is long and loud!

1. Always preheat the oven before baking desserts. There's nothing worse for dessert fruit fillings than to start the baking process in a cold oven.

2. Many of these desserts can be served warm with a dollop of ice cream, or cold with a spoonful of reduced-calorie whipped topping. Just be sure to let the dessert sit on a wire rack for at least 5 minutes before serving. This will give it enough time so that it will scoop out of the pan more easily.

3. Freeze any leftovers in single-serve microwavable freezer containers. Then, when you want to serve "freshly" made desserts, simply remove the lid and microwave on HIGH for about 30 to 60 seconds. Spoon the dessert into a pretty dessert dish and no one will be the wiser—unless you tell them!

4. Your fruit desserts are going to be only as good as the ingredients you use. So, if you're using overripe apples, they're almost guaranteed to make the dessert mushy. If you use under-ripe bananas, the taste won't be as good as if you'd used bananas that were ripe but not overripe. If you use rock-hard peaches, no amount of baking will soften them. If you want your desserts to garner compliments for the cook, use the best-looking fruit you can find!

5. Measure carefully. A bit too much flour or oats in the crumb topping, and it will turn out dry. On the other hand, if you "eyeball" the margarine and use more than you should, your crumb topping will bake into crumb bricks instead of a tender topping.

6. If a recipe calls for apple-pie spice or pumpkin-pie spice, you can get by using ground cinnamon instead. Your dessert won't be quite as scrumptious as it could be because of the missing spices that are part of the blends, but it will still taste fine.

Cherry-Almond Cobbler Criss Cross

Better than a cherry pie to whet your kids' appetites is this visually enticing cherry dessert that offers a peek into the treasure that lies beneath the strips of crust! If you've never made a criss cross delight, here's your chance to make everybody happy.

❤ Serves 8

> *2 (20-ounce) cans sugar-free cherry pie filling*
> *½ cup + 1 tablespoon SPLENDA Granular ☆*
> *½ teaspoon almond extract*
> *¼ cup slivered almonds*
> *1 refrigerated unbaked 9-inch piecrust*

Preheat oven to 415 degrees. Spray a 7-by-11-inch biscuit pan with butter-flavored cooking spray. In a large bowl, combine cherry pie filling, ½ cup Splenda, and almond extract. Stir in almonds. Spread mixture evenly into prepared pan. Unfold piecrust and let set for 5 minutes. Cut into 8 strips. Using 4 longer strips, evenly arrange strips lengthwise over pie filling. Arrange 4 remaining strips crosswise over top. Lightly spray top with butter-flavored cooking spray, and sprinkle remaining 1 tablespoon Splenda over top. Bake for 25 to 30 minutes. Place pan on a wire rack and let set for at least 10 minutes. Divide into 8 servings.

HINTS: 1. If you can't find purchased sugar-free cherry pie filling, use Grandma JO's Fruit Pie Filling.
2. Criss cross strips for an even more impressive look, if desired.

Each serving equals:

HE: 1 Bread • 1 Fruit • ¾ Fat • 14 Optional Calories

205 Calories • 9 gm Fat • 2 gm Protein • 29 gm Carbohydrate • 117 mg Sodium • 10 mg Calcium • 2 gm Fiber

DIABETIC EXCHANGES: 1 Starch • 1 Fruit • 1 Fat

Cherry Upside-Down Dessert

Don't be surprised if friends and family start turning cartwheels and somersaults when they hear that this topsy-turvy treat is on the menu! Why put the fruit on the bottom of a baked dessert? One taste will make it deliciously clear that baking the fruit that way produces a gorgeously "grilled" flavor!   ☻   Serves 8

> 1½ teaspoons almond extract ☆
> 1 (20-ounce) can sugar-free cherry pie filling
> ¼ cup reduced-calorie margarine ☆
> 1½ cups reduced-fat biscuit baking mix
> ¾ cup SPLENDA Granular
> ⅔ cup fat-free half & half
> ¼ cup slivered almonds

Preheat oven to 350 degrees. Spray a 9-by-9-inch cake pan with butter-flavored cooking spray. Stir ½ teaspoon almond extract into can with cherry pie filling. Evenly spoon cherry-pie-filling mixture into prepared cake pan. Drop 4 teaspoons margarine by ½ teaspoonful evenly over cherry-pie-filling mixture. In a large bowl, combine baking mix and Splenda. Add half & half, remaining 2 tablespoons + 2 teaspoons margarine, and remaining 1 teaspoon almond extract. Mix gently to combine. Spoon batter evenly over top. Sprinkle almonds evenly over all. Bake for 18 to 22 minutes. Place pan on a wire rack and let set for at least 10 minutes. Divide into 8 servings.

HINT: If you can't find purchased sugar-free cherry pie filling, use Grandma JO's Fruit Pie Filling.

Each serving equals:

HE: 1 Bread • 1 Fat • ½ Fruit • ¼ Protein • ¼ Slider • 1 Optional Calorie

183 Calories • 7 gm Fat • 3 gm Protein • 27 gm Carbohydrate • 366 mg Sodium • 53 mg Calcium • 2 gm Fiber

DIABETIC EXCHANGES: 1 Starch • 1 Fat • ½ Fruit

Daddy's Bread Pudding

What daughter doesn't want to please her father, especially when she can honor his memory with a dish that's a favorite for both? My dad dearly loved cherries, chocolate, and bread pudding, so this version is a love story in every bite!   ❍   Serves 6

¼ cup cornstarch ☆
1 cup nonfat dry milk powder ☆
1 cup SPLENDA Granular ☆
3 cups water ☆
1½ teaspoons brandy extract ☆
1 (20-ounce) can sugar-free cherry pie filling
9 slices reduced-calorie white bread, torn into pieces
¼ cup unsweetened cocoa powder
1 tablespoon reduced-calorie margarine

Preheat oven to 350 degrees. Spray an 8-by-8-inch baking dish with butter-flavored cooking spray. In a large saucepan, combine 2 tablespoons cornstarch, ⅓ cup dry milk powder, ½ cup Splenda, and 1½ cups water. Cook over medium heat until mixture starts to thicken, stirring constantly using a wire whisk. Remove from heat. Stir in 1 teaspoon brandy extract and cherry pie filling. Add bread pieces. Mix gently to combine. Evenly spread mixture into prepared baking dish. Bake for 35 to 40 minutes. Place baking dish on a wire rack. Meanwhile, in a medium saucepan, combine remaining 2 tablespoons cornstarch, remaining ⅔ cup dry milk powder, remaining ½ cup Splenda, remaining 1½ cups water, and cocoa powder. Cook over medium heat until mixture thickens and starts to boil, stirring constantly using a wire whisk. Remove from heat. Add remaining ½ teaspoon brandy extract and margarine. Mix well to combine. Cut bread pudding into 6 servings. For each serving, place 1 serving of bread pudding on a dessert plate and drizzle about ¼ cup warm chocolate mixture over top.

HINT: If you can't find purchased sugar-free cherry pie filling, use Grandma JO's Fruit Pie Filling.

Each serving equals:

HE: ¾ Bread • ½ Fat-Free Milk • ½ Fruit • ¼ Fat • ½ Slider • 4 Optional Calories

194 Calories • 2 gm Fat • 9 gm Protein • 35 gm Carbohydrate • 270 mg Sodium • 183 mg Calcium • 3 gm Fiber

DIABETIC EXCHANGES: 1½ Starch • ½ Fat-Free Milk • ½ Fruit

Country Baked Pudding

Creamy, sweet, with a true old-fashioned taste, this delicious dessert is "like Grandma used to make"! The good news: Today's grandmas *and* grandkids can make this treat together.

◑ Serves 8

> 1½ cups water
> 2 tablespoons cornstarch
> 1½ cups SPLENDA Granular ☆
> ¼ cup reduced-calorie margarine ☆
> 2 teaspoons vanilla extract ☆
> 5 to 6 drops yellow food coloring
> ½ teaspoon ground cinnamon
> ½ cup fat-free half & half
> 2 tablespoons fat-free sour cream
> ¼ teaspoon table salt
> 1 cup + 2 tablespoons all-purpose flour
> 1 teaspoon baking powder
> ½ cup seedless raisins
> ¼ cup chopped walnuts

Preheat oven to 350 degrees. Spray a 9-by-9-inch cake pan with butter-flavored cooking spray. In a medium saucepan, bring water to a boil. Stir in cornstarch, 1 cup Splenda, 2 tablespoons margarine, and 1 teaspoon vanilla extract. Continue cooking for 4 to 5 minutes, or until mixture starts to thicken, stirring often. Remove from heat. Stir in yellow food coloring and cinnamon. Pour into prepared cake pan. In a large bowl, combine remaining 2 tablespoons margarine, remaining ½ cup Splenda, half & half, sour cream, salt, and remaining 1 teaspoon vanilla extract. Mix well to combine using a wire whisk. Stir in flour and baking powder using a sturdy spoon. Fold in raisins and walnuts. Spoon mixture by heaping tablespoons over liquid mixture in cake pan. Do not stir or spread. Bake for 25 to 30 minutes, or until topping is set and liquid is bubbly. Place pan on a wire rack and let set for at least 5 minutes. Divide into 8 servings.

Each serving equals:

HE: 1 Fat • ¾ Bread • ½ Fruit • ¼ Slider • 18 Optional Calories

182 Calories • 6 gm Fat • 3 gm Protein • 29 gm Carbohydrate • 219 mg Sodium • 63 mg Calcium • 1 gm Fiber

DIABETIC EXCHANGES: 1 Fat • 1 Starch • ½ Fruit

Fruit Baked Apples

For a blissfully better baked apple, try this citrusy-spicy mélange of flavors, warmed to a winning combination! You'll keep the doctor away with each and every bite.   ☺   Serves 6

> 1 cup unsweetened apple juice
> ½ cup diet lemon-lime soda pop
> 1 tablespoon cornstarch
> ½ cup SPLENDA Granular
> ¼ teaspoon apple-pie spice
> ⅔ cup dried mixed fruit, chopped
> 1 tablespoon reduced-calorie margarine
> 6 small tart baking apples

Preheat oven to 350 degrees. Spray an 8-by-8-inch baking dish with butter-flavored cooking spray. In a medium saucepan, combine apple juice, soda pop, cornstarch, Splenda, and apple-pie spice. Stir in chopped mixed fruit. Cook over medium heat until mixture thickens and starts to boil, stirring constantly. Remove from heat. Add margarine. Mix well to combine. Set aside. Remove cores from apples, cutting to but not through bottoms. Peel 1 inch of apple peel from around top of apples. Place apples in prepared baking dish. Fill centers with fruit filling. Evenly spoon remaining fruit filling over tops of filled apples. Bake for 45 to 55 minutes, or until apples are tender. Place baking dish on a wire rack and let set for at least 5 minutes.

HINT: This dessert is good warm or cold.

Each serving equals:

HE: 2 Fruit • ¼ Fat • 12 Optional Calories

133 Calories • 1 gm Fat • 1 gm Protein • 30 gm Carbohydrate • 51 mg Sodium • 17 mg Calcium • 3 gm Fiber

DIABETIC EXCHANGES: 2 Fruit • ½ Fat

Old-Time Apple Betty

How can I describe an apple betty to you? It's a baked fruit sensation without a traditional crust like a pie, and it's topped with a crumbly, crunchy topping! It's been beloved of country cooks for decades, and this version is spectacularly easy to prepare.

○ Serves 8

> 2 (20-ounce) cans sugar-free apple-pie filling
> 1 teaspoon apple-pie spice
> ½ cup SPLENDA Granular ☆
> 1½ cups graham-cracker crumbs
> ⅓ cup reduced-calorie margarine

Preheat oven to 375 degrees. Spray a 7-by-11-inch biscuit pan with butter-flavored cooking spray. In a large bowl, combine apple-pie filling, apple-pie spice, and 2 tablespoons Splenda. Evenly spoon mixture into prepared pan. In a medium bowl, combine graham-cracker crumbs and remaining 6 tablespoons Splenda. Add margarine. Mix well using a pastry blender or 2 forks until mixture becomes crumbly. Sprinkle crumb mixture evenly over apple mixture. Bake for 25 to 30 minutes. Place pan on a wire rack and let set for at least 10 minutes. Divide into 8 servings.

HINT: Instead of using purchased apple-pie filling, you can prepare 2 recipes of Grandma JO's Apple Pie Filling.

Each serving equals:

HE: 1 Bread • 1 Fruit • 1 Fat • 6 Optional Calories

125 Calories • 5 gm Fat • 1 gm Protein • 19 gm Carbohydrate • 193 mg Sodium • 5 mg Calcium • 1 gm Fiber

DIABETIC EXCHANGES: 1 Starch • 1 Fruit • 1 Fat

Mom's Old-Fashioned Apple Crisp

The ingredients may sound like breakfast, but this dazzling dessert is ideal any time of day (or night)! Depending on which apples are featured in your local farmer's market, you can experiment to find the ones you love best. ☻ Serves 6

> 6 cups (6 medium) tart cooking apples, cored, peeled, and
> sliced
> 1 cup Splenda Granular ☆
> 1½ teaspoons ground cinnamon
> ½ cup quick oats
> 6 tablespoons all-purpose flour
> ¼ cup reduced-calorie margarine

Preheat oven to 350 degrees. Spray an 8-by-8-inch baking dish with butter-flavored cooking spray. Evenly arrange apples in prepared baking dish. Sprinkle ½ cup Splenda and cinnamon evenly over apples. In a medium bowl, combine oats, flour, and remaining ½ cup Splenda. Add margarine. Mix well using a pastry blender or 2 forks until mixture becomes crumbly. Sprinkle crumb mixture evenly over apples. Lightly spray top with butter-flavored cooking spray. Bake for 30 to 35 minutes, or until apples are tender and topping is light golden brown. Place baking dish on a wire rack and let set for at least 10 minutes. Divide into 6 servings.

Each serving equals:

HE: 1 Fruit • 1 Fat • ⅔ Bread • 16 Optional Calories

160 Calories • 4 gm Fat • 2 gm Protein • 29 gm Carbohydrate • 91 mg Sodium • 15 mg Calcium • 2 gm Fiber

DIABETIC EXCHANGES: 1 Fruit • 1 Fat • ½ Starch

Grande Strawberry Rhubarb Crisp

Talk about perfect pairings, and you can't do better than strawberries and rhubarb! Each brings out the very best in the other, and there just isn't a better way to know spring has arrived than to serve this to your loved ones.   ◐   Serves 6

> 1 cup quick oats
> 6 tablespoons reduced-fat biscuit baking mix
> 1½ cups SPLENDA Granular ☆
> 1 teaspoon ground cinnamon
> ¼ cup reduced-calorie margarine
> 3 tablespoons cornstarch
> 1 (4-serving) package sugar-free strawberry gelatin
> ½ cup water
> 3 cups chopped fresh or frozen rhubarb, thawed and drained
> 3 cups frozen unsweetened strawberries, thawed and undrained

Preheat oven to 350 degrees. Spray an 8-by-8-inch baking dish with butter-flavored cooking spray. In a large bowl, combine oats, baking mix, ½ cup Splenda, and cinnamon. Add margarine. Mix well using a pastry blender or 2 forks until mixture becomes crumbly. Pat half of crumb mixture into prepared baking dish. In a medium saucepan, combine cornstarch, dry gelatin, remaining 1 cup Splenda, and water. Stir in rhubarb and strawberries. Cook over medium heat for 15 minutes, or until rhubarb softens, stirring often. Evenly spoon hot mixture over crumb crust. Sprinkle remaining crumb mixture evenly over top. Bake for 30 to 35 minutes. Place baking dish on a wire rack and let set for at least 5 minutes. Divide into 6 servings.

Each serving equals:

HE: 1 Bread • 1 Fat • ½ Fruit • ½ Vegetable • ½ Slider • 5 Optional Calories

205 Calories • 5 gm Fat • 4 gm Protein • 36 gm Carbohydrate • 220 mg Sodium • 89 mg Calcium • 5 gm Fiber

DIABETIC EXCHANGES: 1 Starch • 1 Fat • 1 Fruit

Lemon Coconut Crisp

I love to surprise my readers by including some unexpected ingredients in my recipes, and this one is no exception! When I test recipes, I sometimes have to "think outside the box" to find just the right tastes and textures . . . like the saltine crackers in this sweet dessert.   ☯   Serves 8

1½ cups SPLENDA Granular ☆
6 tablespoons reduced-calorie margarine ☆
14 small saltine crackers made into fine crumbs
1 cup all-purpose flour
¼ cup flaked coconut
¾ teaspoon table salt ☆
½ teaspoon baking soda
2 tablespoons cornstarch
1 cup diet lemon lime soda pop
2 eggs, or equivalent in egg substitute
½ cup lemon juice
½ teaspoon coconut extract

Preheat oven to 350 degrees. In a large bowl, combine ¾ cup Splenda and 5 tablespoons margarine. Add cracker crumbs, flour, coconut, ½ teaspoon salt, and baking soda. Mix gently just to combine. Pat half of mixture into an 8-by-8-inch baking dish. Bake for 10 minutes. Place baking dish on a wire rack and let set while preparing filling. In a medium saucepan, combine remaining ¾ cup Splenda, cornstarch, and ¼ teaspoon salt. Stir in soda pop. Cook over medium heat for 4 to 5 minutes, or until mixture thickens and starts to boil, stirring constantly. Remove from heat. In a small bowl, lightly beat eggs with a wire whisk. Add ¼ cup hot filling mixture to eggs, then return egg mixture to saucepan. Continue cooking over medium heat until mixture comes to a boil, stirring constantly. Remove from heat. Stir in lemon juice and coconut extract. Spoon mixture evenly over partially cooled crust. Sprinkle remaining crumb mixture over top. Bake for 25 to 35 minutes, or until top is golden brown. Place baking dish on a wire rack and allow to cool completely. Refrigerate for at least 1 hour. Divide into 8 servings.

Each serving equals:

HE: 1 Bread • 1 Fat • ¼ Protein • ¼ Slider • 8 Optional Calories

170 Calories • 6 gm Fat • 4 gm Protein • 25 gm Carbohydrate • 488 mg Sodium • 12 mg Calcium • 1 gm Fiber

DIABETIC EXCHANGES: 1½ Starch • 1 Fat

Apple Cinnamon Cobbler

When apples bake, they produce a remarkable sweet juice that seems to bring the entire dish together. This old-fashioned cobbler brims with terrifically tender fruit, gloriously moist and impossible to refuse! ☻ Serves 6

> *1 cup SPLENDA Granular ☆*
> *1 cup + 2 tablespoons all-purpose flour ☆*
> *1 teaspoon apple-pie spice ☆*
> *6 cups (6 medium) cored, peeled and sliced tart cooking*
> *apples*
> *2 tablespoons water*
> *1½ teaspoons baking powder*
> *¼ teaspoon table salt*
> *¼ cup reduced-calorie margarine*
> *1 egg, or equivalent in egg substitute*
> *¼ cup fat-free half & half*
> *½ teaspoon vanilla extract*

Preheat oven to 375 degrees. Spray an 8-by-8-inch baking dish with butter-flavored cooking spray. In a large saucepan, combine ¾ cup Splenda, 2 tablespoons flour, and ¾ teaspoon apple-pie spice. Add apples and water. Mix well to combine. Cook over medium heat for 6 to 8 minutes, or just until apples are tender, stirring occasionally. Evenly spoon apple mixture into prepared baking dish. In a large bowl, combine remaining 1 cup flour, 2 tablespoons Splenda, baking powder, and salt. Add margarine. Mix well using a pastry blender or 2 forks until mixture becomes crumbly. Stir in egg, half & half, and vanilla extract. Drop mixture by tablespoon to form 6 mounds. Lightly spray top with butter-flavored cooking spray. In a small bowl, combine remaining ¼ teaspoon apple-pie spice and remaining 2 tablespoons Splenda. Evenly sprinkle mixture over top. Bake for 18 to 20 minutes, or until topping is golden brown. Place baking dish on a wire rack and let set for at least 5 minutes. Divide into 6 servings.

Each serving equals:

HE: 1 Bread • 1 Fruit • 1 Fat • ¼ Slider • 4 Optional Calories

205 Calories • 5 gm Fat • 4 gm Protein • 36 gm Carbohydrate • 315 mg Sodium • 87 mg Calcium • 3 gm Fiber

DIABETIC EXCHANGES: 1 Starch • 1 Fruit • 1 Fat

Raspberry Pear Cobbler

Fat-free dairy products, especially the sour cream, transform this beautifully basic fruit dessert into a feast for the eyes and taste buds! We can usually get ripe, fresh pears all year round, and whether you use fresh raspberries or frozen, I believe you'll be thrilled with the result. ❂ Serves 6

1½ cups fresh or frozen raspberries
2 cups peeled and chopped fresh pears
¾ cup SPLENDA Granular ☆
2 tablespoons cornstarch
1 egg, or equivalent in egg substitute
½ cup fat-free sour cream
¼ cup fat-free milk
2 tablespoons reduced-calorie margarine
1 cup + 2 tablespoons all-purpose flour
1 teaspoon baking powder
¼ teaspoon table salt

Preheat oven to 375 degrees. Spray an 8-by-8-inch baking dish with butter-flavored cooking spray. In a large bowl, gently combine raspberries, chopped pears, ¼ cup Splenda, and cornstarch. Spoon mixture evenly into prepared baking dish. In another large bowl, combine egg, remaining ½ cup Splenda, sour cream, milk, and margarine. Mix well using a wire whisk. Add flour, baking powder, and salt. Mix well using a sturdy spoon. Drop mixture by tablespoon to form 6 mounds. Bake for 22 to 26 minutes, or until light golden brown. Place baking dish on a wire rack and let set for at least 5 minutes. Divide into 6 servings.

Each serving equals:

HE: 1 Bread • 1 Fruit • ½ Fat • ½ Slider • 14 Optional Calories

199 Calories • 3 gm Fat • 5 gm Protein • 38 gm Carbohydrate • 253 mg Sodium • 101 mg Calcium • 4 gm Fiber

DIABETIC EXCHANGES: 1½ Starch, 1 Fruit • ½ Fat

Hawaiian Pineapple Cobbler

Head to Maui, in your mouth at least, with this abundance of tropical sunshine and sweetness in every bite! Why should only residents of those faraway islands feast on that most passionate fruit, the pineapple?   ☻   Serves 6

> 1 cup + 2 tablespoons reduced-fat biscuit baking mix ☆
> 1½ cups SPLENDA Granular ☆
> 3 (8-ounce) cans pineapple chunks, packed in fruit juice,
>   drained, 2 tablespoons liquid reserved
> ¼ cup reduced-calorie margarine
> 1 egg, or equivalent in egg substitute
> 1 teaspoon coconut extract
> 2 tablespoons flaked coconut

Preheat oven to 350 degrees. Spray an 8-by-8-inch baking dish with butter-flavored cooking spray. In a large bowl, combine 6 tablespoons baking mix and 1 cup Splenda. Add pineapple and reserved pineapple liquid. Mix well to combine. Spread pineapple mixture evenly into prepared baking dish. In a large bowl, combine remaining ½ cup Splenda, margarine, and egg using a wire whisk. Stir in remaining ¾ cup baking mix and coconut extract. Drop batter by tablespoonful to form 6 mounds. Lightly spray top with butter-flavored cooking spray. Sprinkle coconut evenly over top. Bake for 25 to 30 minutes, or until top is golden brown. Place baking dish on a wire rack and let set for at least 5 minutes. Divide into 6 servings.

Each serving equals:

HE: 1 Bread • 1 Fruit • 1 Fat • ½ Slider • 1 Optional Calorie

206 Calories • 6 gm Fat • 4 gm Protein • 34 gm Carbohydrate • 368 mg Sodium • 41 mg Calcium • 1 gm Fiber

DIABETIC EXCHANGES: 1 Starch • 1 Fruit • 1 Fat

Classic Cherry Cobbler

When you see the word "classic," you know it means something good that has endured over time. This dessert is traditional in the very best sense, meaning worthy of celebrating again and again!

● Serves 6

> 1 (14.5-ounce) can tart cherries, packed in water, drained,
>   ½ cup liquid reserved
> ½ cup water
> 2 tablespoons cornstarch
> ¾ cup SPLENDA Granular ☆
> 4 to 6 drops red food coloring (optional)
> ½ teaspoon almond extract
> 1 cup + 2 tablespoons all-purpose flour
> 1½ teaspoons baking powder
> ½ teaspoon table salt
> 3 tablespoons reduced-calorie margarine
> ½ cup fat-free half & half

Preheat oven to 400 degrees. Spray an 8-by-8-inch baking dish with butter-flavored cooking spray. In a medium saucepan, combine reserved cherry liquid, water, cornstarch, and ½ cup Splenda. Stir in cherries and red food coloring (if desired). Cook over medium heat until mixture thickens and starts to boil, stirring often and being careful not to crush cherries. Remove from heat. Stir in almond extract. Spoon hot cherry mixture into prepared baking dish. In a medium bowl, combine flour, remaining ¼ cup Splenda, baking powder, and salt. Add margarine. Mix well using a pastry blender or 2 forks until mixture becomes crumbly. Stir in half & half. Spoon mixture evenly over cherry mixture. Lightly spray top with butter-flavored cooking spray. Bake for 16 to 20 minutes, or until filling is hot and bubbly and topping is golden brown. Place baking dish on a wire rack and let set for at least 10 minutes. Divide into 6 servings.

Each serving equals:

HE: 1 Bread • ¾ Fat • ⅔ Fruit • ¼ Slider • 14 Optional Calories

167 Calories • 3 gm Fat • 4 gm Protein • 31 gm Carbohydrate • 396 mg Sodium • 91 mg Calcium • 1 gm Fiber

DIABETIC EXCHANGES: 1 Starch • 1 Fat • 1 Fruit

Rhubarb Cobbler Dessert

Wow, you may think, *that's a lot of Splenda in one dish*—but rhubarb needs lots of sweetening to bring out its delectable and unique flavor! When we taste-tested this dish, we couldn't decide which was better—the fruity part or the scrumptious, sweet dough topping.

☻ Serves 8

> *6 cups finely chopped rhubarb*
> *3 cups SPLENDA Granular ☆*
> *1½ cups reduced-fat biscuit baking mix ☆*
> *¼ teaspoon ground cinnamon*
> *⅓ cup reduced-calorie margarine*
> *1 egg, or equivalent in egg substitute*
> *¼ cup fat-free half & half*
> *1 teaspoon baking powder*

Preheat oven to 350 degrees. Spray a 9-by-13-inch cake pan with butter-flavored cooking spray. In a large bowl, combine rhubarb, 2 cups Splenda, ¼ cup baking mix, and cinnamon. Evenly spoon mixture into prepared cake pan. In a large bowl, combine remaining 1 cup Splenda, margarine, egg, and half & half using a wire whisk. Stir in remaining 1¼ cups baking mix and baking powder using a sturdy spoon. Pour mixture evenly over rhubarb mixture. Bake for 25 to 30 minutes. Place pan on a wire rack and let set for at least 10 minutes. Divide into 8 servings.

Each serving equals:

HE: 1 Bread • 1 Fat • ¾ Vegetable • ½ Slider • 8 Optional Calories

190 Calories • 6 gm Fat • 4 gm Protein • 30 gm Carbohydrate • 375 mg Sodium • 114 mg Calcium • 2 gm Fiber

DIABETIC EXCHANGES: 2 Starch/Carbohydrate • 1 Fat

Strawberry Rhubarb Cobbler

In May, in May, the lovely month of May, you can serve the first of the strawberries and rhubarb in this sensational dessert. It's just like the winners in a ballroom dance contest: two individuals in perfect harmony! ☻ Serves 6

> 3 cups chopped fresh or frozen rhubarb, thawed
> 3 cups frozen unsweetened strawberries, thawed
> 1¼ cups SPLENDA Granular ☆
> 2 tablespoons cornstarch
> ¼ cup reduced-calorie margarine
> ½ cup fat-free half & half
> 1 cup + 2 tablespoons reduced-fat biscuit baking mix
> 1 teaspoon baking powder
> ½ teaspoon ground cinnamon

Preheat oven to 375 degrees. Spray an 8-by-8-inch baking dish with butter-flavored cooking spray. In a large bowl, combine rhubarb, strawberries, 1 cup Splenda, and cornstarch. Spoon mixture evenly into prepared baking dish. In a large bowl, combine margarine, 2 tablespoons Splenda, and half & half using a wire whisk. In a small bowl, combine baking mix and baking powder. Add baking mix mixture to margarine mixture. Mix well using a sturdy spoon. Drop dough by tablespoonful to form 6 mounds. In a small bowl, combine cinnamon and remaining 2 tablespoons Splenda. Evenly sprinkle cinnamon mixture over top. Bake for 45 to 50 minutes, or until filling is hot and bubbly and topping is baked through. Place baking dish on a wire rack and let set for at least 5 minutes. Divide into 6 servings.

Each serving equals:

HE: 1 Bread • 1 Fat • ½ Fruit • ½ Vegetable • ½ Slider • 1 Optional Calorie

209 Calories • 5 gm Fat • 3 gm Protein • 38 gm Carbohydrate • 452 mg Sodium • 155 mg Calcium • 3 gm Fiber

DIABETIC EXCHANGES: 1½ Starch • 1 Fat • ½ Fruit

Raspberry Orange Crumble

Orange juice has such a wonderfully intense flavor, it takes just a little to add shimmer and sparkle to this cozy baked delight. For a special occasion or just on a day you're glad to be alive, serve this sweet treat and give thanks for all your blessings!

◐ Serves 6

> 4½ cups fresh or frozen unsweetened raspberries, thawed
> 1½ cups SPLENDA Granular ☆
> ¾ cup + 1½ tablespoons reduced-fat biscuit baking mix ☆
> 1 tablespoon unsweetened orange juice
> ¼ cup reduced-calorie margarine

Preheat oven to 375 degrees. Spray an 8-by-8-inch baking dish with butter-flavored cooking spray. In a large bowl, combine raspberries, 1 cup Splenda, 1½ tablespoons baking mix, and orange juice. Spoon fruit mixture into prepared baking dish. In a large bowl, combine remaining ¾ cup baking mix, and remaining ½ cup Splenda. Add margarine. Mix well using a pastry blender or 2 forks until mixture forms coarse crumbs. Sprinkle crumb mixture evenly over top of fruit mixture. Bake for 30 to 35 minutes, or until top is golden brown and fruit mixture starts to bubble. Place baking dish on a wire rack and let set for at least 10 minutes. Divide into 6 servings.

HINT: Good served warm with sugar- and fat-free vanilla ice cream, or cold with Cool Whip Lite. If using, don't forget to count the additional calories.

Each serving equals:

HE: 1 Bread • 1 Fruit • 1 Fat • 17 Optional Calories

168 Calories • 5 gm Fat • 2 gm Protein • 31 gm Carbohydrate • 286 mg Sodium • 34 mg Calcium • 5 gm Fiber

DIABETIC EXCHANGES: 1 Starch • 1 Fruit • 1 Fat

Rhubarb Upside-Down Dessert

Who was the first brave cook to prepare a topsy-turvy dessert that practically yelled "surprise" when it was served? Whoever she or he was, I tip my hat to the chef! ☻ Serves 8

> 4 cups finely chopped fresh or frozen rhubarb, thawed
> 2 cups SPLENDA Granular ☆
> 1 cup miniature marshmallows
> 1/3 cup reduced-calorie margarine
> 2 eggs, or equivalent in egg substitute
> 1/4 cup fat-free half & half
> 1 1/2 cups all-purpose flour
> 2 teaspoons baking powder
> 1/4 teaspoon table salt

Preheat oven to 350 degrees. Spray a 9-inch round cake pan with butter-flavored cooking spray. In a large bowl, combine rhubarb and 1 cup Splenda. Evenly spoon rhubarb mixture into prepared cake pan. Sprinkle marshmallows evenly over top. In a large bowl, combine margarine, remaining 1 cup Splenda, and eggs using a wire whisk. Stir in half & half, flour, baking powder, and salt using a sturdy spoon. Spread batter evenly over rhubarb mixture. Bake for 55 to 60 minutes. Place pan on a wire rack and let set for at least 5 minutes. Loosen edges with a knife and place a serving plate over pan. Invert dessert onto serving plate. Cut into 8 servings.

Each serving equals:

HE: 1 Bread • 1 Fat • 1/2 Vegetable • 1/4 Protein • 1/2 Slider • 8 Optional Calories

193 Calories • 5 gm Fat • 5 gm Protein • 32 gm Carbohydrate • 299 mg Sodium • 132 mg Calcium • 2 gm Fiber

DIABETIC EXCHANGES: 2 Starch/Carbohydrate • 1 Fat

Mocha Cappuccino Pudding Cake Dessert

What makes a perfect pudding cake? Rich flavors, stirred together well, baked until done to a moist and delicious turn! If your idea of heaven is smooth, soft pudding in the midst of a great cake, this could be your lucky day! ● Serves 6

1 cup + 2 tablespoons cake flour ☆
1¾ cups SPLENDA Granular ☆
3 tablespoons unsweetened cocoa powder ☆
2½ teaspoons instant coffee crystals ☆
1 teaspoon ground cinnamon
1½ teaspoons baking powder
½ teaspoon table salt
½ cup fat-free half & half
2 tablespoons reduced-calorie margarine
1½ teaspoons vanilla extract ☆
1 (12-fluid-ounce) can evaporated fat-free milk

Preheat oven to 350 degrees. Spray 6 (12-ounce) ovenproof custard cups with butter-flavored cooking spray and evenly arrange on a baking sheet. In a large bowl, combine 1 cup + 1 tablespoon flour, ¾ cup Splenda, 2 tablespoons cocoa powder, 1½ teaspoons coffee crystals, cinnamon, baking powder, and salt. Add half & half, margarine, and 1 teaspoon vanilla extract. Mix gently just to combine. Evenly spoon batter into prepared custard cups. In a medium bowl, combine evaporated milk, remaining 1 cup Splenda, remaining 1 tablespoon four, remaining 1 tablespoon cocoa powder, remaining 1 teaspoon coffee crystals, and remaining ½ teaspoon vanilla extract. Mix gently using a wire whisk. Evenly spoon about ¼ cup milk mixture over batter in each custard cup. Bake for 18 to 22 minutes, or until center is set and firm to touch. Place custard cups on a wire rack and let set for at least 5 minutes.

Each serving equals:

HE: 1 Bread • ½ Fat-Free Milk • ½ Fat • ½ Slider • 6 Optional Calories

191 Calories • 3 gm Fat • 7 gm Protein • 34 gm Carbohydrate • 449 mg Sodium • 251 mg Calcium • 1 gm Fiber

DIABETIC EXCHANGES: 1½ Starch/Carbohydrate • ½ Fat-Free Milk • ½ Fat

Southern Banana Pudding

Some desserts seem to belong to a particular region of our beautiful country, even when they are enjoyed from coast to coast! This soft, sweet pudding seems to me to recall lazy Sunday afternoons sitting on the verandah and dreaming of the good old days.

○ Serves 6

> 1 (12-fluid-ounce) can evaporated fat-free milk
> ½ cup water
> 2 tablespoons cornstarch
> 1 cup SPLENDA Granular ☆
> 1 egg, or equivalent in egg substitute
> 1½ teaspoons vanilla extract ☆
> 18 sugar-free vanilla wafer cookies
> 3 cups (3 medium) sliced bananas ☆
> 3 egg whites

Preheat oven to 350 degrees. Spray an 8-by-8-inch baking dish with butter-flavored cooking spray. In a medium saucepan, combine evaporated milk, water, cornstarch, and ¾ cup Splenda. Stir in egg and 1 teaspoon vanilla extract. Cook over medium heat until mixture thickens and starts to boil, stirring constantly with a wire whisk. Remove from heat. Evenly arrange cookies in prepared baking dish. Layer half the banana slices over cookies. Spoon half of pudding mixture over bananas. Repeat layers with bananas and pudding. In a medium bowl, beat egg whites with an electric mixer on HIGH until soft peaks form. Add remaining ¼ cup Splenda and remaining ½ teaspoon vanilla extract. Continue beating until stiff peaks form. Spread meringue mixture evenly over pudding mixture, being sure to seal to edges of baking dish. Bake for 10 to 15 minutes, or until light brown. Place baking dish on a wire rack and let set for at least 10 minutes. Serve warm, or refrigerate until ready to serve.

HINTS: 1. To prevent bananas from turning brown, mix with 1 teaspoon lemon juice or sprinkle with Fruit Fresh.
2. Egg whites beat best at room temperature.

Each serving equals:

HE: 1 Fruit • ½ Fat-Free Milk • ⅓ Protein • ¾ Slider • 17 Optional Calories

220 Calories • 4 gm Fat • 8 gm Protein • 38 gm Carbohydrate • 160 mg Sodium • 169 mg Calcium • 2 gm Fiber

DIABETIC EXCHANGES: 1 Fruit • 1 Starch • ½ Fat-Free Milk

Lemon-Meringue Pudding Cups

If a true lemon-meringue pie seems too challenging, why not dip your culinary "toe" in the water and stir up these mini-meringues? You've probably got everything you need on hand right now, especially if you love lemony soda pop as much as I do!

◎ Serves 4

> 1 cup SPLENDA Granular ☆
> 3 tablespoons cornstarch
> 1 cup diet lemon-lime soda pop
> 1 egg yolk
> 1 tablespoon + 1 teaspoon reduced-calorie margarine
> ¼ cup lemon juice
> 2 to 3 drops yellow food coloring
> 3 egg whites
> ¼ teaspoon vanilla extract

Preheat oven to 350 degrees. Spray 4 (8-ounce) ovenproof custard cups with butter-flavored cooking spray, and evenly arrange on a baking sheet. In a medium saucepan, combine ¾ cup Splenda and cornstarch. Gradually stir in soda pop. Cook over MEDIUM-HIGH heat until mixture thickens and starts to boil, stirring constantly using a wire whisk. Lower heat and simmer for 2 minutes, stirring often. Remove from heat. Place egg yolk in a large bowl. Stir ½ cup hot filling mixture into egg yolk. Add yolk mixture to filling mixture. Mix well to combine using a wire whisk. Return saucepan to heat and continue cooking for 2 minutes, stirring constantly. Stir in margarine, lemon juice, and food coloring. Evenly spoon mixture into prepared custard cups. In a medium bowl, beat egg whites with an electric mixer until soft peaks form. Add remaining ¼ cup Splenda and vanilla extract. Continue beating until stiff peaks form. Spread meringue mixture evenly over filling mixture in custard cups, being sure to seal to edges. Bake for 8 to 10 minutes, or until meringue starts to turn golden brown. Place custard cups on a wire rack and let set for 30 minutes. Refrigerate for at least 1 hour.

HINT: Egg whites beat best at room temperature.

Each serving equals:

HE: ½ Fat • ¼ Protein • ½ Slider • 17 Optional Calories

91 Calories • 3 gm Fat • 3 gm Protein • 13 gm Carbohydrate • 95 mg Sodium • 9 mg Calcium • 0 gm Fiber

DIABETIC EXCHANGES: 1 Starch • ½ Fat

Aaron's Hot Fudge Pudding Cake

"All kids love pudding cake," my grandson Aaron insisted as we were working together in the kitchen one afternoon. "Especially with hot fudge!" I bet this recipe will prove him right at your house—with kids of all ages! ☉ Serves 8

> 1¾ cups SPLENDA Granular ☆
> 1 cup all-purpose flour
> ½ cup unsweetened cocoa powder ☆
> 2 teaspoons baking powder
> ¼ teaspoon table salt
> ½ cup fat-free half & half
> ⅓ cup reduced-calorie margarine
> 1½ teaspoons vanilla extract
> 1¼ cups hot water
> 1 cup reduced-calorie whipped topping

Preheat oven to 350 degrees. In a large bowl, combine ¾ cup Splenda, flour, ¼ cup cocoa powder, baking powder, and salt. Add half & half, margarine, and vanilla extract. Mix gently just to combine. Evenly pour batter into an ungreased 9-by-9-inch cake pan. In a small bowl, combine remaining 1 cup Splenda and remaining ¼ cup cocoa powder. Sprinkle mixture evenly over batter. Pour hot water evenly over top. Do Not Stir. Bake for 27 to 32 minutes, or until center is almost set. Place pan on a wire rack and let set for 10 minutes. Evenly spoon mixture into 8 dessert dishes and spoon sauce from bottom of pan evenly over each. Garnish with whipped topping.

Each serving equals:

HE: 1 Fat • ⅔ Bread • ½ Slider • 13 Optional Calories

145 Calories • 5 gm Fat • 3 gm Protein • 22 gm Carbohydrate • 264 mg Sodium • 71 mg Calcium • 2 gm Fiber

DIABETIC EXCHANGES: 1 Fat • 1 Starch/Carbohydrate

Apple Cranberry Meringue Dessert

I love doing the unexpected, surprising my family with new flavor sensations and intriguing combos. This dish is a true original, a tart-sweet blend of fruits coupled with the delicate froth of meringue. ☻ Serves 6

½ cup reduced-calorie cranberry juice cocktail
¼ cup water
2 tablespoons cornstarch
1½ cups SPLENDA Granular ☆
1½ cups whole cranberries
1 (20-ounce) can sugar-free apple-pie filling
¼ teaspoon ground cinnamon
6 egg whites
1 teaspoon vanilla extract

Preheat oven to 400 degrees. Spray an 8-by-8-inch baking dish with butter-flavored cooking spray. In a medium saucepan, combine cranberry juice cocktail, water, cornstarch, and 1 cup Splenda. Add cranberries. Mix well to combine. Cover and cook over medium heat for 8 to 10 minutes, or until cranberries soften, stirring occasionally. Remove from heat. Stir in apple-pie filling and cinnamon. Spoon hot mixture evenly into prepared baking dish. Bake for 10 minutes. Meanwhile, in a large bowl, beat egg whites with an electric mixer until soft peaks form. Add remaining ½ cup Splenda and vanilla extract. Continue beating until stiff peaks form. Spread meringue mixture evenly over hot fruit, being sure to seal to edges of baking dish. Bake for 7 minutes or until meringue starts to turn golden brown. Place baking dish on a wire rack and let set for 30 minutes. Refrigerate for at least 1 hour. Divide into 6 servings.

HINT: Egg whites beat best at room temperature.

Each serving equals:

HE: 1 Fruit • ⅓ Protein • ¼ Slider • 14 Optional Calories

96 Calories • 0 gm Fat • 4 gm Protein • 20 gm Carbohydrate • 68 mg Sodium • 7 mg Calcium • 2 gm Fiber

DIABETIC EXCHANGES: 1 Fruit • ½ Other Carbohydrate

Cherry Chocolate Dessert

What's more cheerful than a bowl full of cherries? Two kinds of cherries in a dish that also features chocolate! My son James, the biggest cherry fan in the family, thought this was outstanding.

● Serves 12

2 (1-ounce) unsweetened chocolate squares
⅓ cup reduced-calorie margarine ☆
¾ cup SPLENDA Granular ☆
¾ cup + 2 tablespoons quick oats ☆
1¼ cups reduced-fat biscuit baking mix ☆
1 (20-ounce) can sugar-free cherry pie filling
1 (14.5-ounce) can tart red cherries, packed in water, drained
½ teaspoon brandy extract
¼ cup mini chocolate chips

Preheat oven to 350 degrees. Spray a 9-by-13-inch cake pan with butter-flavored cooking spray. In a medium saucepan, combine chocolate squares, 4 tablespoons margarine, and ¼ cup Splenda. Cook over low heat until mixture is melted, stirring constantly. Remove from heat. Stir in ¾ cup oats, ¾ cup baking mix, and ¼ cup Splenda. Pat mixture into bottom of prepared cake pan. Bake for 10 minutes. Meanwhile, in a large bowl, combine pie filling, tart red cherries, and brandy extract. Evenly spread mixture over baked crust. In a small bowl, combine remaining ½ cup baking mix, remaining 2 tablespoons oats, and remaining ¼ cup Splenda. Add remaining 2 tablespoons margarine. Mix well using a pastry blender or 2 forks until mixture resembles coarse crumbs. Stir in chocolate chips. Sprinkle crumb mixture evenly over top of cherry mixture. Continue baking for 34 to 38 minutes. Place pan on a wire rack and let cool for 15 minutes. Refrigerate for at least 1 hour. Cut into 12 servings.

HINT: If you can't find purchased sugar-free cherry pie filling, use Grandma JO's Fruit Pie Filling.

Each serving equals:

HE: ¾ Bread • ¾ Fat • ⅓ Fruit • ½ Slider • 6 Optional Calories

175 Calories • 7 gm Fat • 3 gm Protein • 25 gm Carbohydrate • 223 mg Sodium • 26 mg Calcium • 3 gm Fiber

DIABETIC EXCHANGES: 1 Starch • 1 Fat • ½ Fruit

Holiday Fudge Torte

Just as we put our best festive apparel on when December rolls around, so too do we want to celebrate with a culinary present to everyone at the table! This utterly decadent delight makes a terrific finale to any big gathering you have planned.

☻ Serves 12

> 1 cup + 2 tablespoons cake flour
> ¾ cup SPLENDA Granular
> ¼ cup unsweetened cocoa powder
> 1½ teaspoons instant coffee crystals
> ¾ teaspoon baking soda
> ¼ teaspoon table salt
> ⅓ cup reduced-calorie margarine
> ¾ cup fat-free sour cream
> 2 eggs, or equivalent in egg substitute
> ½ teaspoon vanilla extract
> 1 recipe Grandma JO's Chocolate Glaze
> ¼ cup chopped walnuts

Preheat oven to 350 degrees. Spray bottom of a 9-inch spring-form pan with butter-flavored cooking spray. In a large bowl, combine flour, Splenda, cocoa powder, coffee crystals, baking soda, and salt. Add margarine, sour cream, eggs, and vanilla extract. Mix gently using a wire whisk until well blended. Pour batter evenly into springform pan. Bake for 18 to 22 minutes, or until a toothpick inserted in center comes out clean. Place pan on wire rack, remove sides, and let set for 10 minutes. Prepare Grandma JO's Chocolate Glaze and drizzle over slightly cooled chocolate layer. Evenly sprinkle walnuts over top. Refrigerate for at least 1 hour. Cut into 12 servings.

HINT: Recipe for Grandma JO's Chocolate Glaze appears in the last chapter.

Each serving equals:

HE: 1 Fat • ½ Bread • ¼ Protein • ½ Slider • 9 Optional Calories

155 Calories • 7 gm Fat • 4 gm Protein • 19 gm Carbohydrate • 231 mg Sodium • 38 mg Calcium • 1 gm Fiber

DIABETIC EXCHANGES: 1½ Starch/Carbohydrate • 1 Fat

Candy Bar Shortcakes

Imagine this scenario: you're baking up a basic shortcake recipe when your favorite peanutty-and-chocolate candy bar accidentally falls into the batter. Wait, didn't Freud say that there are NO accidents? That must mean this outrageous recipe was meant to be!

❤ Serves 6

> 1 cup + 2 tablespoons reduced-fat biscuit baking mix
> ¼ cup SPLENDA Granular
> ⅓ cup nonfat dry milk powder
> ¼ cup reduced-fat peanut butter
> 2 tablespoons fat-free sour cream
> 1 teaspoon vanilla extract
> ⅓ cup water
> ¼ cup mini chocolate chips
> ¼ cup chopped dry-roasted peanuts

Preheat oven to 415 degrees. Spray 6 (8-ounce) ovenproof custard cups with butter-flavored cooking spray. In a large bowl, combine baking mix, Splenda, and dry milk powder. Add peanut butter, sour cream, vanilla extract, and water. Mix gently just to combine. Fold in chocolate chips and peanuts. Evenly spoon batter into prepared custard cups. Arrange custard cups on a baking sheet. Bake for 10 to 12 minutes, or until a toothpick inserted in the center comes out clean. Place custard cups on a wire rack and let set for 5 minutes. Carefully remove shortcakes from custard cups.

HINT: Good served warm with a scoop of sugar- and fat-free vanilla or chocolate ice cream, a drizzle of sugar-free chocolate syrup, and a dollop of reduced-calorie whipped topping. Also good served cold with sliced peaches. If using either, be sure to count the additional calories.

Each serving equals:

HE: 1 Bread • 1 Protein • 1 Fat • ½ Slider • 10 Optional Calories

238 Calories • 10 gm Fat • 7 gm Protein • 30 gm Carbohydrate •
353 mg Sodium • 85 mg Calcium • 2 gm Fiber

DIABETIC EXCHANGES: 1½ Starch/Carbohydrate • 1½ Fat • ½ Meat

Perfect Pies

and Cheesecakes

A friend recently sent me this wonderful quotation from a *Saturday Night Live* sketch starring the character Jack Handy: "When you die, if you get a choice between going to regular heaven or pie heaven, choose pie heaven. It might be a trick, but if it's not, mmmmmmmm, boy." Has he ever got it right! Pie heaven would be a pretty fabulous place—pie for breakfast, pie for lunch, pie for snacktime, and pie for supper! I don't recommend living in pie heaven in this lifetime, but make sure that you put pie on the menu often—you'll get a little taste of pie heaven!

Not too many comedians perform culinary comedy, but I enjoy the food funnies I find from time to time. Here's another one that I rewrote slightly to fit my needs: "How do you make love stay? Tell love you are serving a Healthy Exchanges cheesecake for dinner. Love will stay!"

For a taste of pie heaven, choose from *Decadent Fudgy Brownie Pie*, *Piña Colada Custard Pie*, *Mixed Berry Streusel Pie*, or *Rhubarb Raspberry Meringue Pie*. For cheesecake good enough to make love stay, try *Key West Cheesecake*, *Chocolate Chip Mint Cheesecake*, *Maple Pecan Cheesecake*, or *Spectacular Raspberry Cheesecake*.

Pie and Cheesecake Baking Tips

Pies used to be considered the measure of a great baker, and times haven't changed all that much. But here's the good news: If you follow these baking tips, you'll be the pie baker of your wildest dreams in no time at all!

1. I'm not going to ask you to make your piecrusts from scratch—after all, I usually don't myself! However, I am suggesting that whatever brand of refrigerated piecrusts you purchase, place the piecrust on the counter for 15 to 20 minutes BEFORE you place it in the pie plate. Why, you wonder? This makes the crust much more pliable, and it will go into your pie plate much easier than if you try to arrange a cold crust in the plate.

2. Your pie-baking process will go ever so much smoother if you do any necessary food preparation before assembling the pie. For example, separating eggs, slicing fruit, toasting nuts, or making crumbs out of graham crackers. And be sure to preheat the oven!

3. To help prevent a soggy bottom crust, place the pie in the lower third of the oven for baking, and immediately put the pie plate on a wire rack as soon as it comes out of the oven. The reasons for these suggestions are that the heat is usually the hottest the lower you bake in the oven, and by placing the pie on the wire rack you are allowing for even air circulation, so that the heat from the bottom crust disappears into thin air and isn't forced to go upward into the crust itself.

4. Choosing the proper pie plate goes a long way toward ensuring good baked crusts. Don't use shiny metal pie pans, because they can cause the bottom crust to turn out soggy. Instead, use either a standard glass or a dull metal pie plate. You can save the shiny metal pie pans for making Grandma JO's Graham Cracker Piecrust (see the last chapter).

5. To prevent a crust from over-browning, cover the outside piecrust loosely with foil *or* purchase a piecrust ring created specifically to fit over the crust only of the pie.

6. For double-crusted pies, if you place a piece of elbow macaroni in the center of the top crust, it will act as a chimney and allow the steam to escape from the filling. You can also purchase little ceramic "pie birds" for this purpose. Fruit pies need to bubble in the center to be properly cooked, so don't worry about the steam that puffs out of your pie's chimney!

7. I place a pizza pan under my pie plate when I'm baking fruit pies, so if some of the filling should happen to boil over the crust, the pan will catch it and I won't have to clean my oven nearly as often.

8. Custard pies are done if the center part of the pie that isn't quite firm is less than the size of a quarter. An easy way to test is to insert a table knife near (but not at) the center of the filling. If it comes out clean, the pie is done.

9. Weather can affect your success (or lack of) when making meringues. High humidity can result in a gooey meringue. For best results, make meringues on sunny, low-humidity days or in an air-conditioned kitchen.

10. Make sure both your mixing bowl and the beaters of your electric mixer are completely clean and thoroughly dry before using. Any remaining food specks or moisture really can affect the outcome.

11. When separating eggs for meringue, be sure they are at least one day old and very cold. This makes them separate much more easily. However, be sure to let the egg whites set long enough to come to room temperature before beating, which will produce a higher volume from the whites.

12. Before adding Splenda to the meringue mixture, beat the egg whites to a soft-peak stage first. Always add the Splenda to the egg whites gradually while you continue beating, until the Splenda is completely dissolved. The egg whites should be glossy and stiff, but not dry.

13. When spreading the meringue onto the pie before baking, be sure to spread it completely to the edge to "seal" the filling like a top piecrust would.

14. For best results, cool the baked meringue pie slowly on a wire rack and away from drafts. Then place the cooled pie into the refrigerator for at least an hour. The pie will hold its shape and volume better this way.

15. Meringue pies cut much more easily if your sharp knife is dipped in hot water before you start to cut.

16. For custard-type pies, place the pie plate with the crust already in it into the oven *before* filling. After placing the pie plate in the oven, evenly pour the filling into it. Don't try to carry the prefilled pie from the counter to the oven for fear that you'll spill half the filling before you ever make it to the oven.

17. All of my pies serve 8. This is to ensure that people concerned about diabetes, heart issues, or weight loss don't get too much of a good thing. To make even slices, cut the pie in half, turn it 90 degrees, and cut it in half again. Then cut each quarter in half. Be sure to use a sturdy, sharp knife for cutting, and use a pointed pie spatula for lifting the pie wedge from the pie plate. And remember that the first slice of pie is almost never perfect in appearance!

18. Almost every pie is at its best when eaten no more than 2 to 4 hours after it's been taken out of the oven. However, if you are not going to serve it this fast (or if you have leftovers for another day), cover the pie and refrigerate it for up to 24 hours. The exception to this is fruit pies. To store them, cover and keep them at room temperature, and keep them no longer than a day. If you won't be able to use your leftover pie pieces this fast, place the pie slices on a baking sheet, put them in the freezer, and sharp-freeze them for 2 hours. Then place each piece in its own individual resealable freezer bag, write on the outside

what kind of pie it is and the date you froze it, then place the individual pieces in the freezer. The next time you want "homemade" pie for dessert, remove the number of pieces you need for the meal *just* before you eat, remove them from the freezer bags, and arrange on dessert plates. By the time you are finished with your meal, the slices will be thawed and waiting for you!

19. When preparing cheesecakes, remember that fat-free cream cheese has more water than regular cream cheese. If you beat it with an electric mixer, you will release the water and your filling will be soft and runny. Instead, use a sturdy spoon and stir the cream cheese for 45 to 60 seconds, or until it softens. Then use a good wire whisk to incorporate the other ingredients into the filling.

20. Because fat-free cream cheese does not have the "buffering" effect of all the fat that regular cream cheese does, your finished product may develop thin cracks on the top. After cooling, just cover it with a thin layer of reduced-calorie whipped topping and no one will be the wiser!

21. Buy the best springform pan you can find. You will thank yourself for years to come when the bottom and sides retain their shape and the spring latch that closes the sides remains strong!

22. Use either your hand protected in a Zip-loc sandwich bag or a small measuring cup to press the crumb-crust mixture firmly into the bottom of the springform pan.

23. Don't overbake cheesecakes! Bake only until the center of the cheesecake still has a slight "jiggle" and isn't quite firm yet, while the sides look a bit dry. Don't fret that the center isn't done, as the cheesecake will continue to bake as it cools and the center will firm up.

24. Set a kitchen timer for the time suggested for cooling, and don't remove the sides of the springform pan until the timer rings! If you remove them too soon, the cheesecake

sides may not stay firm on the serving plate, and if you remove them too late, the cheesecake may start to pull away from the edges and begin to crack. To remove the cheesecake from the pan, first run a warm, wet cloth over the outside. Next, run a table knife between the cheesecake and the pan, being careful not to scrape the pan or nick the cheesecake. Unbuckle the pan and remove the sides. I leave the bottom of the pan on my cheesecake and just place it on my serving plate. However, if you wish to remove the metal bottom, use a long, sharp knife and run it between the bottom of the cheesecake and the pan. Be sure to have your serving plate handy to slide the cheesecake onto.

25. Cheesecakes are always better if they are covered and refrigerated for at least 6 hours before serving. And always store leftovers in the refrigerator.

26. A straight-edged, thin-bladed knife works best when cutting cheesecakes. It helps to prevent the cheesecake from clumping and sticking to the knife. Don't use a serrated knife. Also, try to avoid dragging the filling down as you slice, so the pieces remain nice and firm. Dip the knife into hot water and wipe it dry after each cut and you'll have perfect pieces of cheesecake to place on serving plates.

Blueberry Crumble Pie

A two-crust pie is pretty, I admit it, but to me there is nothing more appealing to the eye than the crunchy crust of a crumble! (Can you say that three times fast?) Make sure you use quick oats, not the old-fashioned kind, for this recipe. ☺ Serves 8

> 1 refrigerated unbaked 9-inch piecrust
> 3 cups fresh or frozen unsweetened blueberries
> ¼ cup water
> 1¼ cups SPLENDA Granular ☆
> 2 tablespoons quick tapioca
> 4½ tablespoons graham-cracker crumbs
> ¼ cup quick oats
> 2 tablespoons reduced-calorie margarine

Preheat oven to 375 degrees. Place piecrust in a 9-inch pie plate and flute edges. Prick bottom and sides with tines of a fork. Bake for 8 minutes. Meanwhile, in a medium saucepan, combine blueberries, water, 1 cup Splenda, and tapioca. Cook over medium heat until mixture starts to bubble, stirring occasionally. Lower heat and simmer while crust bakes, stirring often. Evenly pour hot blueberry filling into partially baked piecrust. Place piecrust on a wire rack while preparing topping. In a medium bowl, combine graham-cracker crumbs, oats, and remaining ¼ cup Splenda. Add margarine. Mix well using a pastry blender or 2 forks until mixture becomes crumbly. Sprinkle crumb mixture evenly over blueberry mixture. Continue baking for 18 to 22 minutes, or until filling is bubbly and top is golden brown. Place pie on a wire rack and allow to cool completely. Cut into 8 servings.

HINTS: 1. Piecrust works best if left to set at room temperature for at least 15 minutes before using.

2. To keep piecrust from getting too brown, protect it with either a piecrust shield or strip of aluminum foil.

Each serving equals:

HE: 1⅓ Bread • ¾ Fat • ½ Fruit • ¼ Slider • 5 Optional Calories

209 Calories • 9 gm Fat • 1 gm Protein • 31 gm Carbohydrate • 152 mg Sodium • 6 mg Calcium • 2 gm Fiber

DIABETIC EXCHANGES: 1½ Starch • 1 Fat • ½ Fruit

Mixed Berry Streusel Pie

If you've got a Fourth of July party to go to, here's a gorgeous dessert that everyone would gladly applaud! This blend of berries offers some real culinary fireworks in every delicious bite.

❍ Serves 8

> *1 refrigerated unbaked 9-inch piecrust*
> *3 cups fresh or frozen red raspberries, thawed*
> *3 cups fresh or frozen blueberries, thawed*
> *1½ cups SPLENDA Granular ☆*
> *¾ cup reduced-fat biscuit baking mix ☆*
> *¼ teaspoon ground nutmeg*
> *2 tablespoons reduced-calorie margarine*
> *¼ cup chopped walnuts*

Preheat oven to 375 degrees. Place piecrust in a 9-inch pie plate and flute edges. In a large bowl, combine raspberries and blueberries. Stir in 1 cup Splenda, ¼ cup baking mix, and nutmeg. Evenly spoon fruit mixture into prepared piecrust. In a medium bowl, combine remaining ½ cup Splenda and remaining ½ cup baking mix. Add margarine. Mix well using a pastry blender or 2 forks until mixture becomes crumbly. Stir in walnuts. Sprinkle crumb mixture evenly over fruit mixture. Bake for 15 minutes. Lower oven temperature to 350 degrees and continue baking for 30 minutes, or until filling is bubbly and top is golden brown. Place pie plate on a wire rack and allow to cool completely. Refrigerate for at least 2 hours. Cut into 8 servings.

HINT: Piecrust works best if left to set at room temperature for at least 15 minutes before using.

Each serving equals:

HE: 1½ Bread • 1 Fruit • 1 Fat • ½ Slider • 10 Optional Calories

267 Calories • 11 gm Fat • 4 gm Protein • 38 gm Carbohydrate • 266 mg Sodium • 30 mg Calcium • 3 gm Fiber

DIABETIC EXCHANGES: 1½ Starch • 1½ Fat • 1 Fruit

Apple Crisp Pie

What's more American than apple-pie? Not much, but this cozy and flavorful old-fashioned pie is a delectable throwback to the good old days, when moms would stir up a simple topping for a one-crust pie. Yummy!　❂　Serves 8

> 1 refrigerated unbaked 9-inch piecrust
> 6 cups (6 medium) cored, peeled and thinly sliced cooking
>   apples
> ¼ cup unsweetened apple juice
> 1 tablespoon lemon juice
> 1½ cups SPLENDA Granular ☆
> 8 tablespoons all-purpose flour ☆
> 1½ teaspoons apple-pie spice
> ½ cup quick oats
> 2 tablespoons + 2 teaspoons reduced-calorie margarine

Preheat oven to 375 degrees. Place piecrust in a 9-inch deep-dish pie plate and flute edges. In a large bowl, combine apples, apple juice, and lemon juice. Add 1 cup Splenda, 2 tablespoons flour, and apple-pie spice. Mix gently just to combine. Evenly spoon apple mixture into prepared piecrust. In a medium bowl, combine oats, remaining 6 tablespoons flour, and remaining ½ cup Splenda. Add margarine. Mix well using a pastry blender or 2 forks until mixture becomes crumbly. Sprinkle crumb mixture evenly over apple mixture. Bake for 40 to 45 minutes, or until filling is bubbly and top is golden brown. Place pie plate on a wire rack and allow to cool completely. Cut into 8 servings.

HINT: Piecrust works best if left to set at room temperature for at
    least 15 minutes before using.

Each serving equals:

HE: 1 ½ Bread • 1 Fruit • 1 Fat • ¼ Slider • 1 Optional Calorie

245 Calories • 9 gm Fat • 2 gm Protein • 39 gm Carbohydrate • 147 mg Sodium •
10 mg Calcium • 3 gm Fiber

DIABETIC EXCHANGES: 1½ Starch • 1½ Fat • 1 Fruit

Pear Cranberry Crumb Pie

When I set out to create a new recipe, I think about flavors, of course. But I also contemplate how different textures will combine. This pie asks two less familiar fruits to join hands and create a dessert delight for the whole family to love. ☻ Serves 8

1 refrigerated unbaked 9-inch piecrust
½ cup reduced-fat biscuit baking mix ☆
¼ cup fat-free half & half
1 teaspoon ground cinnamon
1¼ cups SPLENDA Granular ☆
3½ cups peeled and chopped Bartlett pears
1 cup chopped fresh or frozen cranberries
2 tablespoons + 2 teaspoons reduced-calorie margarine

Preheat oven to 375 degrees. Place piecrust in a 9-inch pie plate and flute edges. In a large bowl, combine 2 tablespoons baking mix, half & half, and cinnamon. Stir in 1 cup Splenda. Add pears and cranberries. Mix well to combine. Evenly spoon fruit mixture into prepared piecrust. In a medium bowl, combine remaining 6 tablespoons baking mix and remaining ¼ cup Splenda. Add margarine. Mix well using a pastry blender or 2 forks until mixture becomes crumbly. Sprinkle crumb mixture evenly over fruit mixture. Bake for 15 minutes. Lower oven temperature to 350 degrees. Continue baking for 40 to 45 minutes, or until filling is bubbly and top is golden brown. Place pie plate on a wire rack and allow to cool completely. Cut into 8 servings.

HINT: Piecrust works best if left to set at room temperature for at least 15 minutes before using.

Each serving equals:

HE: 1½ Bread • 1 Fruit • 1 Fat • 19 Optional Calories

238 Calories • 10 gm Fat • 2 gm Protein • 35 gm Carbohydrate •
243 mg Sodium • 23 mg Calcium • 3 gm Fiber

DIABETIC EXCHANGES: 1½ Starch • 1½ Fat • 1 Fruit

Impossible French Apple Pie

Remember how they say in the Army: "The difficult we do immediately; the impossible takes a little longer"? This pie isn't more time-consuming to prepare than others; what's remarkable about it is how your batter "blossoms" in the heat of the oven into a splendid dessert. Ooh-la-la! ☻ Serves 8

> 4 cups (4 medium) cored, peeled and thinly sliced Granny
>   Smith apples
> 1½ cups SPLENDA Granular ☆
> 1½ teaspoons apple-pie spice
> ¾ cup fat-free milk
> 2 eggs, or equivalent in egg substitute
> ¼ cup reduced-calorie margarine ☆
> 1½ cups reduced-fat biscuit baking mix ☆
> ¼ cup chopped walnuts

Preheat oven to 325 degrees. Spray a 9-inch pie plate with butter-flavored cooking spray. In a large bowl, combine apples, 1 cup Splenda, and apple-pie spice. Evenly spoon apple mixture into prepared pie plate. In same bowl, combine milk, eggs, 1 tablespoon margarine, and ½cup baking mix. Mix well using a wire whisk. Evenly pour mixture over apple mixture. In a medium bowl, combine remaining 1 cup baking mix and remaining ½ cup Splenda. Add remaining 3 tablespoons margarine. Mix well using a pastry blender or 2 forks until mixture becomes crumbly. Stir in walnuts. Sprinkle crumb mixture evenly over top. Bake for 55 to 60 minutes, or until a knife inserted in center comes out clean. Place pie plate on a wire rack and allow to cool completely. Cut into 8 servings.

Each serving equals:

HE: 1 Bread • 1 Fat • ½ Fruit • ⅓ Protein • ¼ Slider • 6 Optional Calories

212 Calories • 8 gm Fat • 5 gm Protein • 30 gm Carbohydrate • 357 mg Sodium • 70 mg Calcium • 2 gm Fiber

DIABETIC EXCHANGES: 1 Starch • 1 Fruit • 1 Fat

Grandma's Old-Fashioned Pumpkin Pie

Gobbling turkey isn't the only way to celebrate the arrival of the holiday season! Why not bring true warmth and joy into your home by serving up a classic pie with just a few modern-day tricks? You'll be so glad you did! ☕ Serves 8

> 1 refrigerated unbaked 9-inch piecrust
> 1 (12-fluid-ounce) can evaporated fat-free milk
> ⅓ cup nonfat dry milk powder
> ¾ cup SPLENDA Granular
> 1½ teaspoons pumpkin-pie spice
> 2 eggs, or equivalent in egg substitute
> 1 (15-ounce) can solid-pack pumpkin

Preheat oven to 425 degrees. Place piecrust in a deep dish 9-inch pie plate and flute edges. In a large bowl, combine evaporated milk and dry milk powder. Stir in Splenda, pumpkin-pie spice, and eggs. Add pumpkin. Mix well to combine. Evenly pour mixture into prepared piecrust. Bake for 15 minutes. Lower oven temperature to 350 degrees. Continue baking for 40 to 50 minutes, or until a knife inserted in the center comes out clean. Place pie plate on a wire rack and allow to cool completely. Cut into 8 servings.

HINT: Piecrust works best if left to set at room temperature for at least 15 minutes before using.

Each serving equals:

HE: 1 Bread • ½ Fat-Free Milk • ½ Fat • ½ Vegetable • ¼ Protein • 9 Optional Calories

208 Calories • 8 gm Fat • 7 gm Protein • 27 gm Carbohydrate • 195 mg Sodium • 175 mg Calcium • 2 gm Fiber

DIABETIC EXCHANGES: 1 Starch/Carbohydrate • 1 Fat • ½ Fat-Free Milk

Chocolate Chip Pie

We've got loads of cookies and even ice cream flavors that feature that baking "celebrity," the irresistible chocolate chip! Now this icon has a pie to call its own—a marvelous dessert that shines a beautiful light on this old baking reliable. Don't make cookies tonight— prepare a pie instead!   ☻   Serves 8

> ¼ cup reduced-calorie margarine
> ¼ cup unsweetened applesauce
> 2 eggs, or equivalent in egg substitute
> 1 cup SPLENDA Granular
> ½ cup all-purpose flour
> ½ cup mini chocolate chips
> 1 purchased chocolate crumb piecrust

Preheat oven to 325 degrees. In a large bowl, combine margarine, applesauce, eggs, and Splenda. Mix well using a wire whisk. Add flour. Mix gently just to combine using a sturdy spoon. Fold in chocolate chips. Evenly spread batter into piecrust. Bake for 38 to 46 minutes, or until a knife inserted in center comes out clean. Place pie on a wire rack and allow to cool completely. Cut into 8 servings.

Each serving equals:

HE: 1¼ Bread • 1 Fat • ¼ Protein • ¾ Slider • 19 Optional Calories

235 Calories • 11 gm Fat • 4 gm Protein • 30 gm Carbohydrate • 187 mg Sodium • 13 mg Calcium • 1 gm Fiber

DIABETIC EXCHANGES: 2 Starch/Carbohydrate • 1½ Fat

Brownie Walnut Pie

Adore brownies rich with crunchy nuts but want a more glamorous presentation? Here's a pie that shines the spotlight on these favorite flavors! It's rich and nutty, dark and sweet, and it's a terrific birthday treat.   ☻   Serves 8

4 eggs or equivalent in egg substitute
¼ cup reduced-calorie margarine
2 tablespoons fat-free half & half
½ cup reduced-fat biscuit baking mix
½ cup unsweetened cocoa powder
1½ cups SPLENDA Granular
1 teaspoon vanilla extract
¼ cup chopped walnuts

Preheat oven to 350 degrees. Spray a 9-inch pie plate with butter-flavored cooking spray. In a large bowl, combine eggs, margarine, and half & half using a wire whisk. Add baking mix, cocoa, Splenda, and vanilla extract. Mix well to combine using a sturdy spoon. Stir in walnuts. Evenly spread batter into prepared pie plate. Bake for 23 to 26 minutes, or until a knife inserted in center comes out clean. Place pie plate on a wire rack and allow to cool completely. Cut into 8 servings.

Each serving equals:

HE: 1 Fat • ⅔ Protein • ⅓ Bread • ¼ Slider • 12 Optional Calories

148 Calories • 8 gm Fat • 5 gm Protein • 14 gm Carbohydrate • 196 mg Sodium • 36 mg Calcium • 2 gm Fiber

DIABETIC EXCHANGES: 1 Fat • 1 Starch/Carbohydrate • ½ Meat

Decadent Fudgy Brownie Pie

Do you remember when the lead woman singer in *Cabaret* waved her green fingernails at someone and said, "Divine decadence, darling"? Liza Minnelli played Sally Bowles in the movie, and she had the right idea about decadence being heavenly, just as this pie is!

◐ Serves 8

> 1 cup reduced-calorie chocolate syrup
> 1 tablespoon + 1 teaspoon reduced-calorie margarine
> 1 recipe Grandma JO's Sweetened Condensed Milk
> 6 tablespoons reduced-fat biscuit baking mix
> ¼ cup SPLENDA Granular
> 2 eggs, or equivalent in egg substitute
> 1 teaspoon vanilla extract
> 1 (6-ounce) purchased chocolate piecrust

Preheat oven to 375 degrees. In a large bowl, combine chocolate syrup, margarine, and Grandma JO's Sweetened Condensed Milk using a wire whisk. Add baking mix, Splenda, eggs, and vanilla extract. Mix well to combine using a sturdy spoon. Evenly pour batter into piecrust. Bake for 35 to 40 minutes, or until center is set. Place pie on a wire rack and allow to cool completely. Cut into 8 servings.

HINT: Recipe for Grandma JO's Sweetened Condensed Milk appears in last chapter.

Each serving equals:

HE: 1¼ Bread • ½ Fat-Free Milk • ½ Fat • ¼ Protein • ½ Slider • 10 Optional Calories

236 Calories • 8 gm Fat • 7 gm Protein • 34 gm Carbohydrate • 282 mg Sodium • 166 mg Calcium • 1 gm Fiber

DIABETIC EXCHANGES: 2 Starch/Carbohydrate • 1 Fat • ½ Fat-Free Milk

Old-Fashioned Custard Pie

It used to be something only very experienced cooks with tons of time on their hands even attempted, but now custard pie can be prepared with perfection (or almost) by just about anyone. This filling is oh-so-rich, it ought to be nicknamed after those Olsen Twins!

● Serves 8

1 refrigerated unbaked 9-inch piecrust
4 eggs, or equivalent in egg substitute
¾ cup SPLENDA Granular
¼ teaspoon table salt
1 (12-fluid-ounce) can evaporated fat-free milk
1 cup fat-free milk
1 tablespoon vanilla extract
¼ teaspoon ground nutmeg

Preheat oven to 425 degrees. Place piecrust in a deep dish 9-inch pie plate and flute edges. In a large bowl, beat eggs with a wire whisk for 1 minute. Stir in Splenda and salt. Add evaporated milk, fat-free milk, and vanilla extract. Mix well to combine. Evenly pour mixture into prepared piecrust. Lightly sprinkle nutmeg over top. Bake for 10 minutes. Lower oven temperature to 350 degrees. Continue baking for 25 to 30 minutes, or until a knife inserted in center comes out clean. Place pie plate on a wire rack and let set for 30 minutes. Refrigerate for at least 1 hour. Cut into 8 servings.

HINT: Piecrust works best if left to set at room temperature for at least 15 minutes before using.

Each serving equals:

HE: 1 Bread • ½ Fat-Free Milk • ½ Protein • ½ Fat • 9 Optional Calories

214 Calories • 10 gm Fat • 8 gm Protein • 23 gm Carbohydrate • 280 mg Sodium • 171 mg Calcium • 1 gm Fiber

DIABETIC EXCHANGES: 1 Starch • 1 Fat • ½ Fat-Free Milk • ½ Meat

Piña Colada Custard Pie

If the drink tastes like nectar, why not turn it into a scrumptious pie? That's what I said when I was stirring up recipes for this chapter. The combination of pineapple and coconut with just a touch of rum flavor will send your taste buds, at least, on an island sojourn!

☻ Serves 8

> 1 cup fat-free half & half
> 1 (8-ounce) can crushed pineapple, packed in fruit juice, undrained
> 1½ teaspoons coconut extract
> 1 teaspoon rum extract
> ½ cup reduced-fat biscuit baking mix
> ½ cup SPLENDA Granular
> 2 eggs, or equivalent in egg substitute
> 1 tablespoon + 1 teaspoon reduced-calorie margarine
> ¼ cup flaked coconut ☆

Preheat oven to 350 degrees. Spray a 9-inch pie plate with butter-flavored cooking spray. In a large bowl, combine half & half, undrained pineapple, coconut extract, and rum extract using a wire whisk. Add baking mix, Splenda, eggs, margarine, and 2 tablespoons coconut. Mix well to combine using a sturdy spoon. Evenly spoon mixture into prepared pie plate. Bake for 10 minutes. Sprinkle remaining 2 tablespoons coconut evenly over top of partially baked pie. Continue to bake for 18 to 22 minutes, or until a knife inserted in center comes out clean. Place pie plate on a wire rack and allow to cool completely. Cut into 8 servings.

Each serving equals:

HE: ⅓ Bread • ¼ Protein • ¼ Fruit • ¼ Fat • ¼ Slider • 15 Optional Calories

108 Calories • 4 gm Fat • 3 gm Protein • 15 gm Carbohydrate • 179 mg Sodium • 44 mg Calcium • 1 gm Fiber

DIABETIC EXCHANGES: 1 Starch/Carbohydrate • ½ Fat

Lemon "Buttermilk" Pie

Wondering what to serve at a summer card party for all of your friends? This luscious, light, and oh-so-lemony pie will win you plenty of applause, but I can't guarantee a winning hand at poker or bridge! If you're wondering where the "buttermilk" is, you're going to make it yourself with the milk powder, water, and lemon juice.   ☻   Serves 8

> 1 refrigerated unbaked 9-inch piecrust
> 1⅓ cups dry milk powder
> 1½ cups water
> ½ cup lemon juice
> 1 tablespoon + 1 teaspoon reduced-calorie margarine
> 1½ cups SPLENDA Granular
> 2 eggs, or equivalent in egg substitute
> 2 tablespoons cornstarch

Preheat oven to 375 degrees. Place piecrust in a deep dish 9-inch pie plate and flute edges. Prick bottom and sides with tines of a fork. Bake for 8 minutes. Place pie plate on a wire rack. Lower oven temperature to 350 degrees. In a medium bowl, combine dry milk powder, water, and lemon juice. Set aside. In a large bowl, combine margarine and Splenda using a wire whisk. Add eggs. Mix well to combine. Stir in cornstarch and milk mixture. Evenly pour mixture into piecrust. Bake for 40 to 45 minutes, or until a knife inserted in center comes out clean. Place pie plate on a wire rack and let set for 30 minutes. Refrigerate for at least 2 hours. Cut into 8 servings.

HINT: Piecrust works best if left to set at room temperature for at least 15 minutes before using.

Each serving equals:

HE: 1 Bread • ¾ Fat • ½ Fat-Free Milk • ¼ Protein • ¼ Slider •
6 Optional Calories

222 Calories • 10 gm Fat • 6 gm Protein • 27 gm Carbohydrate •
215 mg Sodium • 159 mg Calcium • 1 gm Fiber

DIABETIC EXCHANGES: 1½ Fat • 1 Starch • ½ Fat-Free Milk

Oatmeal Maple Pie

Up in Vermont, where sweet maple syrup turns up in nearly every baked dish prepared, this old-fashioned pie would be headed for the state fair! Every bite will remind you just how delicious maple flavor is when coupled with hearty oats. ☽ Serves 8

1 refrigerated unbaked 9-inch piecrust
4 eggs, or equivalent in egg substitute
1 cup SPLENDA Granular
2 tablespoons reduced-calorie margarine
¾ cup fat-free milk
1 teaspoon vanilla extract
½ cup sugar-free maple syrup
3 tablespoons all-purpose flour
¼ cup quick oats
¼ cup flaked coconut

Preheat oven to 350 degrees. Place piecrust in a 9-inch pie plate and flute edges. In a large bowl, combine eggs, Splenda, and margarine using a wire whisk. Stir in milk, vanilla extract, and maple syrup. Add flour and oats. Mix gently just to combine using a sturdy spoon. Fold in coconut. Evenly pour mixture into prepared piecrust. Bake on lowest rack in oven for 40 to 45 minutes, or until a knife inserted in center comes out clean. Place pie plate on a wire rack and allow to cool completely. Cut into 8 servings.

HINT: Piecrust works best if left to set at room temperature for at least 15 minutes before using.

Each serving equals:

HE: 1¼ Bread • 1 Fat • ½ Protein • ½ Slider • 1 Optional Calorie

223 Calories • 11 gm Fat • 6 gm Protein • 25 gm Carbohydrate •
210 mg Sodium • 44 mg Calcium • 1 gm Fiber

DIABETIC EXCHANGES: 2 Fat • 1½ Starch • ½ Meat

Rhubarb Raspberry Meringue Pie

We all learn the "three R's" in school, but I'd like to introduce you to two more "R's" that really make the grade! Rhubarb brings its special tangy tartness to any recipe, while raspberries contribute a wild sweetness that is truly exhilarating. Add a fluffy meringue, and you're ready for any special occasion.   ☺   Serves 8

1 refrigerated unbaked 9-inch piecrust
4 cups chopped fresh or frozen rhubarb, thawed
½ cup + 2 tablespoons water ☆
3 cups frozen unsweetened raspberries, thawed, drained, 2
    tablespoons liquid reserved
2 tablespoons cornstarch
1½ cups SPLENDA Granular ☆
6 egg whites
1 teaspoon coconut extract
2 tablespoons flaked coconut

Preheat oven to 415 degrees. Place piecrust in a 9-inch pie plate and flute edges. Prick bottom and sides with tines of a fork. Bake for 9 to 10 minutes, or until lightly browned. Place pie plate on a wire rack and allow to cool. Meanwhile, in a medium saucepan, combine rhubarb, ½ cup water, and reserved raspberry liquid. Cover and cook over medium heat for 5 minutes, or until rhubarb is tender, stirring occasionally. In a small bowl, combine remaining 2 tablespoons water and cornstarch using a wire whisk. Mix well until it forms a paste. Add cornstarch mixture and 1 cup Splenda to rhubarb mixture. Mix well to combine. Continue cooking for 2 to 3 minutes, stirring constantly. Remove from heat. Stir in raspberries. Evenly spoon hot mixture into cooled piecrust. In a large glass bowl, beat egg whites with an electric mixer on HIGH until soft peaks form. Add remaining ½ cup Splenda and coconut extract. Continue beating on HIGH until stiff peaks form. Evenly spread meringue mixture over filling mixture, being sure to seal to edges of piecrust. Sprinkle coconut evenly over top. Bake for 6 to 8 minutes, or until meringue starts to turn golden brown. Place pie plate on a wire rack and let set for 30 minutes. Refrigerate for at least 2 hours. Cut into 8 servings.

HINTS: 1. Piecrust works best if left to set at room temperature for at least 15 minutes before using.
2. Egg whites beat best at room temperature.
3. Meringue pie cuts easily if you dip a sharp knife in warm water before slicing.

Each serving equals:

HE: 1 Bread • ½ Fruit • ½ Fat • ½ Vegetable • ¼ Protein • ¼ Slider •
10 Optional Calories

200 Calories • 8 gm Fat • 4 gm Protein • 28 gm Carbohydrate • 147 mg Sodium •
66 mg Calcium • 4 gm Fiber

DIABETIC EXCHANGES: 1 Starch/Carbohydrate • 1 Fruit • 1 Fat

Nut Meringue Pie with Chocolate Filling

Meringues look as if they might be way too challenging for the average home cook, but I intend to persuade you to "take the plunge"! If you follow instructions, you can learn to make dazzling desserts like this one with only a little extra effort—and it's well worth the time spent.   ◐   Serves 8

> 6 egg whites
> 2 teaspoons vanilla extract ☆
> ½ teaspoon cream of tartar
> ⅛ teaspoon table salt
> ¾ cup SPLENDA Granular
> ¼ cup chopped walnuts
> ½ cup mini chocolate chips
> 2 tablespoons hot water
> 1½ cups reduced-calorie whipped topping

Preheat oven to 275 degrees. In a large glass bowl, beat egg whites with an electric mixer on HIGH until soft peaks form. Stir in 1 teaspoon vanilla extract, cream of tartar, salt, and Splenda. Continue beating on HIGH until stiff peaks form. Evenly spread meringue mixture in the bottom and up the sides of a 9-inch pie plate. Sprinkle walnuts evenly over top. Bake for 50 to 60 minutes. Place pie plate on a wire rack and let set for 30 minutes. Meanwhile, place chocolate chips in a medium-size microwave-safe bowl. Stir in water and remaining 1 teaspoon vanilla extract. Microwave on HIGH (100% power) for 30 seconds or until chocolate chips are melted. Mix well to combine. Place bowl on a wire rack and let set for 30 minutes. Fold in whipped topping. Evenly spoon chocolate mixture into cooled meringue crust. Refrigerate for at least 2 hours. Cut into 8 servings.

HINTS: 1. Egg whites beat best at room temperature.
2. Meringue pie cuts easily if you dip a sharp knife in warm water before slicing.

Each serving equals:

HE: ⅓ Protein • ¼ Fat • 1 Slider • 11 Optional Calories

131 Calories • 7 gm Fat • 4 gm Protein • 13 gm Carbohydrate • 79 mg Sodium • 9 mg Calcium • 1 gm Fiber

DIABETIC EXCHANGES: 1 Other Carbohydrate • 1 Fat

Easy Baked Cheesecake

Most of my cheesecake recipes don't call for any "oven time," but this one requires that you turn up the heat for a scrumptious delight! You might decide to have a cheesecake tasting competition, where you offer side-by-side tastes of baked versus my chilled style. Wouldn't that be fun? Mm-mm! ◐ Serves 8

> 2 (8-ounce) packages fat-free cream cheese
> 1 cup SPLENDA Granular ☆
> ¼ cup reduced-fat biscuit baking mix
> ½ cup fat-free half & half
> 2 eggs, or equivalent in egg substitute
> 1 tablespoon vanilla extract ☆
> 1 purchased 6-ounce graham-cracker piecrust
> ¾ cup fat-free sour cream

Preheat oven to 325 degrees. In a large bowl, stir cream cheese with a sturdy spoon until softened. Add ¾ cup Splenda, baking mix, half & half, eggs, and 2 teaspoons vanilla extract. Mix well to combine using a wire whisk. Evenly pour mixture into piecrust. Bake for 25 to 35 minutes, or until center is set. Place pie plate on a wire rack and let set for 1 hour. In a small bowl, combine sour cream, remaining ¼ cup Splenda and remaining 1 teaspoon vanilla extract. Evenly spread mixture over cooled cheesecake. Cover and refrigerate for at least 2 hours. Cut into 8 servings.

Each serving equals:

HE: 1¼ Protein • 1 Bread • ¼ Fat • ½ Slider • 17 Optional Calories

226 Calories • 6 gm Fat • 12 gm Protein • 31 gm Carbohydrate •
527 mg Sodium • 215 mg Calcium • 1 gm Fiber

DIABETIC EXCHANGES: 1 Meat • 1 Starch/Carbohydrate • 1 Fat

Key West Cheesecake

If you've ever wondered where Jimmy Buffett's famous "Margaritaville" is, you'll find it on a laid-back South Florida island called Key West! And what goes perfectly with a cold margarita (or Diet Dew)? Why, a luscious lime-flavored cheesecake!

● Serves 12

1 cup + 2 tablespoons graham-cracker crumbs
1 cup + 2 tablespoons SPLENDA Granular ☆
2 tablespoons reduced-calorie margarine
3 (8-ounce) packages fat-free cream cheese
2 eggs
½ cup fat-free sour cream
½ cup lime juice
2 tablespoons cornstarch

Preheat oven to 350 degrees. Spray a 9-inch springform pan with butter-flavored cooking spray. In a medium bowl combine graham-cracker crumbs, 2 tablespoons Splenda, and margarine. Mix well using a pastry blender or 2 forks until mixture becomes crumbly. Press mixture into prepared pan. Bake for 5 minutes. Place pan on a wire rack. Meanwhile, in a large bowl, stir cream cheese with a sturdy spoon until softened. Stir in eggs and sour cream. Add lime juice, cornstarch, and remaining 1 cup Splenda. Mix well using a wire whisk. Evenly pour batter over crust in springform pan. Bake for 40 to 45 minutes, or until center is set. Remove from oven and place on a wire rack, and let set for 1 hour. Cover and refrigerate for at least 3 hours. Run a knife along inside edges of pan. Remove sides. Cut into 12 servings.

Each serving equals:

HE: 1 Protein • ½ Bread • ¼ Fat • ¼ Slider • 13 Optional Calories

131 Calories • 3 gm Fat • 10 gm Protein • 16 gm Carbohydrate •
375 mg Sodium • 181 mg Calcium • 1 gm Fiber

DIABETIC EXCHANGES: 1 Meat • 1 Starch/Carbohydrate

Spectacular Raspberry Cheesecake

Sometimes, it's worth adding a few extra ingredients in order to transform a basic cake into one worthy of a big event, a major occasion—and this is my nominee for the culinary Oscars! It's extra-creamy, super-luscious, and downright decadent in all the right ways. ☻ Serves 12

18 (2½-inch) chocolate graham crackers, made into fine
    crumbs
¼ cup SPLENDA Granular
2 tablespoons reduced-calorie margarine
3 (8-ounce) packages fat-free cream cheese
2 eggs, or equivalent in egg substitute
1 recipe Grandma JO's Sweetened Condensed Milk
¼ cup fat-free sour cream
1 teaspoon vanilla extract
¼ cup mini chocolate chips
1½ cups fresh or frozen unsweetened raspberries
⅔ cup raspberry spreadable fruit
1½ cups reduced-calorie whipped topping
5 to 6 drops red food coloring

Preheat oven to 325 degrees. Spray a 9-inch springform pan with butter-flavored cooking spray. In a medium bowl, combine chocolate graham-cracker crumbs, Splenda, and margarine. Mix well using a pastry blender or 2 forks until mixture becomes crumbly. Press mixture into prepared pan. Bake for 5 minutes. Place pan on a wire rack. Meanwhile, in a large bowl, stir cream cheese with a sturdy spoon until softened. Add eggs and Grandma JO's Sweetened Condensed Milk. Mix well to combine using a wire whisk. Stir in sour cream and vanilla extract. Gently fold in chocolate chips and raspberries using a rubber spatula. Evenly pour batter over crust in springform pan. Bake for 45 to 50 minutes, or until center is set. Remove from oven and place on a wire rack and let set for 30 minutes. Cover and refrigerate for at least 4 hours. Run a knife along inside edges of pan. Remove sides. In a medium bowl, stir spreadable fruit with a spoon to soften. Add whipped topping and red food coloring. Mix gently just to combine. Spread topping mixture evenly over cheesecake. Cut into 12 servings.

HINTS: 1. A self-seal sandwich bag works great for crushing graham crackers.
2. Recipe for Grandma JO's Sweetened Condensed Milk appears in last chapter.

Each serving equals:

HE: 1 Protein • ¾ Fruit • ½ Bread • ¼ Fat • ¼ Slider • 17 Optional Calories

196 Calories • 4 gm Fat • 13 gm Protein • 27 gm Carbohydrate •
397 mg Sodium • 276 mg Calcium • 1 gm Fiber

DIABETIC EXCHANGES: 1 Starch/Carbohydrate • 1 Fruit • 1 Meat • ½ Fat

Pineapple Rum Cheesecake

When the temperature's high and you can't escape the heat, why not pretend you're stranded in the tropics—and sipping a festive rum drink from a coconut shell? (You can often find fun fake ones on sale to make the fantasy more real!) Then cut a piece of this rich and irresistible sun-kissed treasure, and you'll feel as if you've discovered a pirate's treasure buried in all that sand.

☻ Serves 12

> 1¼ cups graham-cracker crumbs
> 1¼ cups SPLENDA Granular ☆
> 2 tablespoons reduced-calorie margarine
> 3 (8-ounce) packages fat-free cream cheese
> 2 eggs, or equivalent in egg substitute
> 1 teaspoon rum extract
> 2 (8-ounce) cans crushed pineapple, packed in fruit juice,
>   drained and ¼ cup liquid reserved
> ½ cup fat-free sour cream
> 2 tablespoons cornstarch
> 1½ cups reduced-calorie whipped topping
> 1 teaspoon coconut extract
> 3 tablespoons flaked coconut

Preheat oven to 325 degrees. Spray a 9-inch springform pan with butter-flavored cooking spray. In a medium bowl, combine graham-cracker crumbs, ¼ cup Splenda, and margarine. Mix well using a pastry blender or 2 forks until mixture becomes crumbly. Press mixture into prepared pan. Set aside. In a large bowl, stir cream cheese with a sturdy spoon until softened. Stir in remaining 1 cup Splenda, eggs, and rum extract. Add pineapple, reserved pineapple liquid, sour cream, and cornstarch. Mix gently just to combine using a wire whisk. Evenly pour batter over crust in springform pan. Bake for 55 to 60 minutes, or until center is set. Remove from oven and place on a wire rack, and let set for 30 minutes. Cover and refrigerate for at least 4 hours. Run a knife along inside edges of pan. Remove sides. In a small bowl, combine whipped topping and coconut extract. Evenly spread topping mixture over cheesecake. Sprinkle coconut evenly over top. Cut into 12 servings.

Each serving equals:

HE: 1 Protein • ½ Bread • ⅓ Fruit • ¼ Fat • ¾ Slider • 2 Optional Calories

189 Calories • 5 gm Fat • 11 gm Protein • 25 gm Carbohydrate • 387 mg Sodium • 180 mg Calcium • 1 gm Fiber

DIABETIC EXCHANGES: 1½ Starch/Carbohydrate • 1 Meat • ½ Fat

Thanksgiving Pumpkin Cheesecake

Determined not to serve the same old pies on Turkey Day this year? Here's my advice for a holiday treat that's perfect—and pumpkin! The hearty orange veggie gives the filling an extra intensity that makes you want to savor each and every bite.   ● Serves 12

1 cup + 2 tablespoons graham-cracker crumbs
6 tablespoons finely chopped pecans ☆
1½ cups SPLENDA Granular ☆
2 tablespoons reduced-calorie margarine
3 (8-ounce) packages fat-free cream cheese
2 eggs, or equivalent in egg substitute
2 tablespoons fat-free half & half
1 tablespoon cornstarch
1 (15-ounce) can solid-pack pumpkin
1½ teaspoons pumpkin-pie spice
2 teaspoons vanilla extract ☆
1 cup fat-free sour cream

Preheat oven to 350 degrees. Spray a 9-inch springform pan with butter-flavored cooking spray. In a medium bowl, combine graham-cracker crumbs, 3 tablespoons pecans, ¼ cup Splenda, and margarine. Mix well using a pastry blender or 2 forks until mixture becomes crumbly. Press mixture into prepared pan. Set aside. In a large bowl, stir cream cheese with a sturdy spoon until softened. Stir in eggs, 1 cup Splenda, half & half, and cornstarch. Mix well to combine. Add pumpkin, pumpkin-pie spice, and 1 teaspoon vanilla extract. Mix well to combine using a wire whisk. Evenly pour batter over crust in springform pan. Bake for 50 to 55 minutes, or until center is set. Remove from oven and place on a wire rack and let set for 1 hour. In a small bowl, combine sour cream, remaining ¼ cup Splenda, and remaining 1 teaspoon vanilla extract. Evenly spread mixture over cooled cheesecake. Sprinkle remaining 3 tablespoons pecans over top. Cover and refrigerate for at least 3 hours. Run a knife along inside edges of pan. Remove sides. Cut into 12 servings.

Each serving equals:

HE: 1 Protein • ¾ Fat • ½ Bread • ⅓ Vegetable • ½ Slider • 5 Optional Calories

182 Calories • 6 gm Fat • 12 gm Protein • 20 gm Carbohydrate • 394 mg Sodium • 206 mg Calcium • 2 gm Fiber

DIABETIC EXCHANGES: 1 Meat • 1 Fat • 1 Starch/Carbohydrate

Cappuccino Cheesecake

Wouldn't it be lovely to sip a cup of fragrant cappuccino at a café in Florence or that city of dreams, Venice? I'd love to, but tonight I've got time for only a dessert delectable enough to transport me (in my dreams) to Italy! This cake is truly a recipe for romance.

◑ Serves 12

> 24 (2½-inch) chocolate graham-cracker squares, made into fine crumbs
> ¼ cup reduced-calorie margarine, melted
> 4 (8-ounce) packages fat-free cream cheese
> 1 cup + 2 tablespoons reduced-calorie chocolate syrup ☆
> ½ cup + 2 tablespoons SPLENDA Granular ☆
> 3 eggs, or equivalent in egg substitute
> ¼ cup fat-free half & half
> 1 teaspoon instant coffee crystals ☆
> ½ teaspoon ground cinnamon
> 2 teaspoons vanilla extract ☆
> 2 cups reduced-calorie whipped topping

Preheat oven to 350 degrees. Reserve ¼ cup chocolate graham-cracker crumbs. In a medium bowl, combine remaining chocolate graham-cracker crumbs and melted margarine. Press mixture into an ungreased 9-inch springform pan. Set aside. In a large bowl, stir cream cheese with a sturdy spoon until softened. Stir in 1 cup chocolate syrup. Add ½ cup Splenda, eggs, and half & half. Mix well to combine using a wire whisk. Fold in ½ teaspoon instant coffee crystals, cinnamon, and 1½ teaspoons vanilla extract. Evenly pour batter over crust in springform pan. Bake for 50 to 55 minutes, or until center is set. Remove from oven and place on a wire rack and let set for 1 hour. In a large bowl, gently combine whipped topping, remaining 2 tablespoons chocolate syrup, remaining 2 tablespoons Splenda, remaining ½ teaspoon instant coffee crystals, and remaining ½ teaspoon vanilla extract. Evenly spread mixture over cooled cheesecake. Sprinkle reserved ¼ cup chocolate graham-cracker crumbs evenly over top. Cover and refrigerate for at least

2 hours. Run a knife along inside edges of pan. Remove sides. Cut into 12 servings.

HINT: If you are a "strong" coffee drinker, you may want to use 2 teaspoons instant coffee crystals.

Each serving equals:

HE: 1½ Protein • ⅔ Bread • ½ Fat • ¾ Slider • 12 Optional Calories

201 Calories • 5 gm Fat • 15 gm Protein • 24 gm Carbohydrate • 599 mg Sodium • 359 mg Calcium • 1 gm Fiber

DIABETIC EXCHANGES: 1½ Meat • 1½ Starch/Carbohydrate

Latte Cheesecake

There was a time, not so long ago, when most Americans had no idea what a latte was, but now this frothy coffee and steamed milk combo is available in nearly every town in the USA! Just as latte drinkers top off their "treat in a cup" with a sprinkle of cinnamon, a touch of chocolate, and a dollop of whipped cream, so too can dessert lovers revel in those flavors in a piece of this cheesecake.

◐ Serves 12

1½ cups graham-cracker crumbs
1 cup SPLENDA Granular ☆
¼ cup reduced-calorie margarine
3 (8-ounce) packages fat-free cream cheese
2 eggs, or equivalent in egg substitute
2 tablespoons cornstarch
¼ teaspoon ground nutmeg
1½ teaspoons vanilla extract
¾ cup fat-free sour cream
⅓ cup cold coffee
1½ cups reduced-calorie whipped topping
⅛ teaspoon ground cinnamon
3 tablespoons mini chocolate chips

Preheat oven to 325 degrees. Spray a 9-inch springform pan with butter-flavored cooking spray. In a medium bowl, combine graham-cracker crumbs, ¼ cup Splenda, and margarine. Mix well using a pastry blender or 2 forks until mixture becomes crumbly. Press mixture into prepared pan. Set aside. In a large bowl, stir cream cheese with a sturdy spoon until softened. Stir in remaining ¾ cup Splenda. Add eggs, cornstarch, nutmeg, and vanilla extract. Mix well to combine using a wire whisk. Fold in sour cream and coffee. Evenly pour batter over crust in springform pan. Bake for 45 to 50 minutes, or until center is set. Remove from oven and place on a wire rack and let set for 30 minutes. Refrigerate for at least 4 hours. Run a knife along inside edges of pan. Remove sides. Spread whipped topping evenly over cheesecake. Sprinkle cinnamon and chocolate chips evenly over top. Cut into 12 servings.

Each serving equals:

HE: 1 Protein • ⅔ Bread • ½ Fat • ¾ Slider • 11 Optional Calories

182 Calories • 6 gm Fat • 10 gm Protein • 22 gm Carbohydrate •
421 mg Sodium • 189 mg Calcium • 1 gm Fiber

DIABETIC EXCHANGES: 1½ Starch/Carbohydrate • 1 Meat • ½ Fat

Chocolate Chip Mint Cheesecake

My friend Barbara told me that her favorite ice cream when she was a little girl was mint chocolate chip, so I wanted to give her a culinary memory of happy days with this fresh and flavorful treat. The next time she visits me in Iowa, I'm putting this on the menu!

● Serves 12

18 (2½-inch) chocolate graham crackers, crushed into fine
    crumbs
½ cup + 2 tablespoons SPLENDA Granular ☆
3 tablespoons reduced-calorie margarine
3 (8-ounce) packages fat-free cream cheese
2 tablespoons cornstarch
2 eggs, or equivalent in egg substitute
¾ cup fat-free sour cream
1 teaspoon mint extract
4 to 6 drops green food coloring
½ cup mini chocolate chips
1½ cups reduced-calorie whipped topping

Preheat oven to 325 degrees. Spray a 9-inch springform pan with butter-flavored cooking spray. In a medium bowl, combine chocolate graham-cracker crumbs, 2 tablespoons Splenda, and margarine. Mix well using a pastry blender or 2 forks until mixture becomes crumbly. Press mixture into prepared pan. Set aside. In a large bowl, stir cream cheese with a sturdy spoon until softened. Stir in remaining ½ cup Splenda, cornstarch, eggs, sour cream, and mint extract using a wire whisk. Add green food coloring. Mix gently just to combine. Fold in chocolate chips using a rubber spatula. Evenly pour batter over crust in springform pan. Bake for 45 to 50 minutes, or until center is set. Remove from oven and place on a wire rack and let set for 30 minutes. Cover and refrigerate for at least 4 hours. Run a knife along inside edges of pan. Remove sides. Spread whipped topping evenly over cheesecake. Cut into 12 servings.

HINT: A self-seal sandwich bag works great for crushing graham crackers.

Each serving equals:

HE: 1 Protein • ½ Bread • ⅓ Fat • 1 Slider • 8 Optional Calories

178 Calories • 6 gm Fat • 11 gm Protein • 20 gm Carbohydrate • 444 mg Sodium • 285 mg Calcium • 1 gm Fiber

DIABETIC EXCHANGES: 1 Meat • 1 Starch/Carbohydrate • 1 Fat

Maraschino Cherry and Chocolate Cheesecake

For their wedding not too many years ago, a young couple decided to order cherry chocolate cheesecakes from a famous Brooklyn, New York, bakery to serve to their guests. "It's what we love best," they told me, which makes perfect sense to me. There will be no pricey shipping charges when you stir up this version of that dreamy dessert. ☻ Serves 12

1 cup + 2 tablespoons graham-cracker crumbs
3 tablespoons unsweetened cocoa powder
1¼ cups SPLENDA Granular ☆
2 tablespoons + 2 teaspoons reduced-calorie margarine
3 (8-ounce) packages fat-free cream cheese
4 eggs, or equivalent in egg substitute
1 tablespoon cornstarch
¼ cup fat-free half & half
1 teaspoon almond extract
12 maraschino cherries ☆
¼ cup mini chocolate chips

Preheat oven to 350 degrees. Spray a 9-inch springform pan with butter-flavored cooking spray. In a medium bowl, combine graham-cracker crumbs, cocoa powder, ¼ cup Splenda, and margarine. Mix well using a pastry blender or 2 forks until mixture becomes crumbly. Press mixture into prepared pan. Set aside. In a large bowl, stir cream cheese with a sturdy spoon until softened. Add eggs, cornstarch, and remaining 1 cup Splenda. Mix well to combine using a wire whisk. Stir in half & half and almond extract. Quarter 8 maraschino cherries. Pat cherries with paper towel to absorb liquid. Gently fold cherry pieces and chocolate chips into cream cheese mixture using a rubber spatula. Evenly pour batter over crust in springform pan. Bake for 45 to 55 minutes, or until center is set. Remove from oven and place on a wire rack and let set for 1 hour. Quarter remaining 4 maraschino cherries. Garnish top of cheesecake with cherry pieces. Cover and refrigerate for at least 2 hours. Remove sides from pan. Cut into 12 servings.

HINT: If desired, drizzle with Grandma JO's Chocolate Glaze. Also good served with a dollop of reduced-calorie whipped topping. If using, don't forget to count the additional calories.

Each serving equals:

HE: 1⅓ Protein • ½ Bread • ⅓ Fat • ½ Slider • 5 Optional Calories

169 Calories • 5 gm Fat • 12 gm Protein • 19 gm Carbohydrate • 453 mg Sodium • 277 mg Calcium • 1 gm Fiber

DIABETIC EXCHANGES: 1½ Meat • 1 Starch/Carbohydrate • ½ Fat

Maple Pecan Cheesecake

Nuts are one of nature's most remarkable gifts—a crunchy-sweet prize hidden beneath a tough exterior! My most favorite nut is the splendid pecan, and I'm so glad that just a few tablespoons impart so much flavor, so I can stir them into a maple-rich cheesecake and really taste them.   ☺   Serves 12

1¼ cups graham-cracker crumbs
1 cup SPLENDA Granular
2 tablespoons reduced-calorie margarine
3 (8-ounce) packages fat-free cream cheese
½ cup sugar-free maple syrup
2 eggs, or equivalent in egg substitute
2 tablespoons cornstarch
½ cup fat-free sour cream
3 tablespoons chopped pecans

Preheat oven to 325 degrees. Spray a 9-inch springform pan with butter-flavored cooking spray. In a medium bowl, combine graham-cracker crumbs, Splenda, and margarine. Mix well using a pastry blender or 2 forks until mixture becomes crumbly. Press mixture into prepared pan. Set aside. In a large bowl, stir cream cheese with a sturdy spoon until softened. Stir in maple syrup and eggs. Add cornstarch and sour cream. Mix gently just to combine using a wire whisk. Evenly pour batter over crust in springform pan. Sprinkle pecans evenly over top. Bake for 40 to 45 minutes, or until center is set. Remove from oven and place on a wire rack, and let set for 30 minutes. Cover and refrigerate for at least 4 hours. Run a knife along inside edges of pan. Remove sides. Cut into 12 servings.

Each serving equals:

HE: 1 Protein • ½ Bread • ½ Fat • ½ Slider • 1 Optional Calorie

152 Calories • 4 gm Fat • 11 gm Protein • 18 gm Carbohydrate •
397 mg Sodium • 181 mg Calcium • 1 gm Fiber

DIABETIC EXCHANGES: 1 Starch/Carbohydrate • 1 Meat • ½ Fat

Splenda Sugar Blend for Baking Beauties

Why mess with something that isn't broken? After all, Splenda is a fantastic sugar substitute, approved by the FDA, shelf-stable, with no aftertaste, so why did the manufacturer produce this hybrid product? Essentially, the Sugar Blends for Baking were created to use in recipes where sugar previously played a more substantial role. For people who want to cut down on their sugar use but not eliminate sugar from their diets, this product offers a delicious compromise that works especially well in recipes calling for a large amount of sugar. The Splenda website quotes Colin Watts, president of McNeil Nutritionals, a division of McNeil-PPC, Inc., saying, "We see this product really changing the way people think about sugar." The site further explains that "SPLENDA® Sugar Blend for Baking contains sugar, which allows consumers to achieve the browning, rising, spreading, and texture that baked goods made with sugar possess. Consumers will only need to use half a cup of SPLENDA® Sugar Blend for Baking to achieve the sweetness of a full cup of sugar."

What kinds of recipes "ask" for SPLENDA Sugar Blend for Baking? Oh, just wait until you try James's Old-Fashioned Blondies, Mom's Angel Food Cake, *and* Becky's Prize-Winning Banana Bread. *You'll be signing up for the school bake sale or inviting your card club for afternoon tea! And for something really special, try using SPLENDA's brown sugar blend to make* Grandma's Cinnamon Rolls *or my truly delightful* Buttermilk Coffee Cake. *You'll be so glad you did!*

Read the following tips to learn more about using this exciting new product, and you'll be ready to experience a new kind of healthy baking.

Splenda Sugar Blends Baking Tips

Please refer to the specific chapters for general baking tips for muffins, cookies, cakes, pies, or desserts. However, there are a few "tricks of the trade" to be aware of when baking with either Splenda Sugar Blend for Baking or Splenda Brown Sugar Blend.

1. Splenda Blends have been specifically created to use with baked goods—especially those in which sugar plays a major role in the finished product. However, the blends also have many more calories and carbs than regular Splenda Granular. For comparison purposes, 1 tablespoon of sugar contains 48 calories, with a whopping 48 grams carbohydrate; 1 tablespoon of Splenda Blend contains 24 calories, with 24 grams of carbohydrate; and 1 tablespoon of Splenda Granular contains only 6 calories, with just 4.5 grams of carbohydrate. That's why I've chosen to focus mostly on Splenda Granular in this book. However, I've created this "blends" chapter for when you occasionally want something really special and a little bit will do.

2. When converting your own recipes to the Splenda Sugar Blends, keep in mind that ½ cup of either of the blends equals 1 cup of sugar or brown sugar. I've already taken this into consideration when I created the recipes in this chapter.

3. Your cookies will spread easier when using the Blends. Your cakes will lightly brown when using the Blends. Your baked goods will rise a bit higher when using the Blends. Why? Because of the sugar that is blended into the Splenda Blends, that's why.

Rolled Sugar Cookies

Love sugar cookies but figure there's no way to make them healthy *and* tasty? Think again! Cookies like these are the reason Splenda's blend for baking was created—and, boy, does it work well. These are lovely to serve with tea when friends drop by.

◐ Serves 16 (2 each)

> ⅔ cup reduced-calorie margarine
> 2 tablespoons fat-free sour cream
> 1 egg, or equivalent in egg substitute
> 1½ teaspoons vanilla extract
> 1½ cups SPLENDA Sugar Blend for Baking
> 2½ cups + 2 tablespoons all-purpose flour
> 1½ teaspoons baking powder
> ¼ teaspoon table salt

In a large bowl, combine margarine, sour cream, egg, and vanilla extract using a wire whisk. Stir in Splenda Sugar Blend for Baking. Add 2½ cups flour, baking powder, and salt. Mix gently to combine using a sturdy spoon. Cover and refrigerate for at least 2 hours. Just before baking, preheat oven to 375 degrees and spray 3 baking sheets with butter-flavored cooking spray. Shape dough into a ball. Sprinkle remaining 2 tablespoons flour evenly over pastry board or counter. Place dough on floured surface and roll out to a ¼-inch thickness. Using a 2-inch cookie cutter, cut into 32 cookies, pressing dough together as necessary. Place cookies on prepared baking sheets. Bake for 10 to 12 minutes, or until bottoms are lightly browned. Remove cookies from baking sheets and cool on wire racks.

HINT: If desired, lightly sprinkle with colored sugar crystals just before baking, or frost with Grandma JO's Frosting Glaze after cooling.

Each serving equals:

HE: 1 Fat • ¾ Bread • ½ Slider • 8 Optional Calories

140 Calories • 4 gm Fat • 2 gm Protein • 24 gm Carbohydrate • 158 mg Sodium • 23 mg Calcium • 0 gm Fiber

DIABETIC EXCHANGES: 1 Fat • 1 Starch

If Prepared with Sugar and Butter:

221 Calories • 9 gm Fat • 2 gm Protein • 33 gm Carbohydrate

John's Homestyle Chocolate Chip Cookies

I got my entire family involved in testing recipes for this book—in this case, I reinvented one of my son-in-law John's particular favorites, the classic chocolate chip cookie, just as he likes it—without nuts but with both kinds of sugar flavor. He told me these were "just perfect," which certainly warmed this mom-in-law's heart!   ❂   Serves 8 (3 each)

⅓ cup reduced-calorie margarine
1 egg, or equivalent in egg substitute
½ cup SPLENDA Sugar Blend for Baking
¼ cup SPLENDA Brown Sugar Blend
1 teaspoon vanilla extract
1½ cups all-purpose flour
½ teaspoon baking soda
¼ teaspoon table salt
½ cup mini chocolate chips

Preheat oven to 350 degrees. Spray 2 baking sheets with butter-flavored cooking spray. In a large bowl, combine margarine and egg using a wire whisk. Stir in Splenda Sugar Blend for Baking, Splenda Brown Sugar Blend, and vanilla extract. In a small bowl, combine flour, baking soda, and salt. Add flour mixture to margarine mixture. Mix gently just to combine using a sturdy spoon. Fold in chocolate chips. Drop batter by full teaspoonful to form 24 cookies. Bake for 11 to 15 minutes, or until lightly browned. Place baking sheets on wire racks and let set for 2 minutes. Remove cookies from baking sheets and continue to cool on wire racks.

HINTS: 1. Use a very, very large mixing bowl to help incorporate air into the margarine, egg, and Splenda mix.
2. To drop cookies onto baking sheet, remove batter from one teaspoon by using another teaspoon, or use a small cookie scoop.

Each serving equals:

HE: 1 Bread • 1 Fat • 1 Slider • 19 Optional Calories

219 Calories • 7 gm Fat • 4 gm Protein • 35 gm Carbohydrate • 253 mg Sodium • 15 mg Calcium • 1 gm Fiber

DIABETIC EXCHANGES: 2 Starch/Carbohydrate • 1 Fat

If Prepared with Sugar, Brown Sugar, and Butter:

300 Calories • 12 gm Fat • 4 gm Protein • 44 gm Carbohydrate

Chocolate Chip Apricot Oatmeal Cookies

What a marvelous mélange of flavors fight for your attention in each and every cookie gem this recipe makes! Who said you can't have it all? In this recipe, it sure seems as if you can!

❂ Serves 12 (2 each)

½ cup reduced-calorie margarine
¾ cup SPLENDA Sugar Blend for Baking
2 tablespoons SPLENDA Brown Sugar Blend
¼ cup unsweetened applesauce
1 egg, or equivalent in egg substitute
¾ cup all-purpose flour
1 teaspoon baking soda
¼ cup graham-cracker crumbs
2 cups quick oats
¾ cup chopped dried apricots
½ cup mini chocolate chips

Preheat oven to 350 degrees. Spray 2 baking sheets with butter-flavored cooking spray. In a large bowl, combine margarine, Splenda Sugar Blend for Baking, and Splenda Brown Sugar Blend using a wire whisk. Stir in applesauce and egg. In a small bowl, combine flour, baking soda, graham-cracker crumbs, and oats. Add flour mixture to margarine mixture. Mix gently just to combine using a sturdy spoon. Fold in apricots and chocolate chips. Drop by tablespoonful onto prepared baking sheets to form 24 cookies. Lightly flatten cookies with the bottom of a glass sprayed with butter-flavored cooking spray. Bake for 10 to 14 minutes. Do Not Overbake. Place baking sheets on wire racks and let set for 2 minutes. Remove cookies from baking sheets and continue to cool on wire racks.

HINT: Best stored in an open container.

Each serving equals:

HE: 1 Bread • 1 Fat • ¾ Fruit • ¾ Slider • 13 Optional Calories

211 Calories • 7 gm Fat • 4 gm Protein • 33 gm Carbohydrate • 215 mg Sodium • 19 mg Calcium • 3 gm Fiber

DIABETIC EXCHANGES: 1 Starch/Carbohydrate • 1 Fat • 1 Fruit

If Prepared with Sugar and Butter:

315 Calories • 15 gm Fat • 4 gm Protein • 41 gm Carbohydrate

Pam's Crunchy Cookies

My daughter-in-law Pam is a busy mom of three boys, but she still finds time to mix up a batch of cookies for the kids. She asked me to create a recipe that incorporated a little brown-sugar flavor along with a family-favorite cereal, Rice Krispies. Now, she tells me, the boys ask for Mom's "special" cookies when they want her to bake something special.   ☻   Serves 12 (3 each)

> ½ cup reduced-calorie margarine
> ¾ cup SPLENDA Sugar Blend for Baking
> 2 tablespoons SPLENDA Brown Sugar Blend
> 1 egg, or equivalent in egg substitute
> 1 teaspoon vanilla extract
> 1¼ cups all-purpose flour
> ½ teaspoon baking powder
> ¼ teaspoon table salt
> 2 cups Rice Krispies cereal

Preheat oven to 375 degrees. Spray baking sheets with butter-flavored cooking spray. In a large bowl, combine margarine, Splenda Sugar Blend for Baking, Splenda Brown Sugar Blend, egg, and vanilla extract using a wire whisk. In a small bowl, combine flour, baking powder, and salt. Add flour mixture to margarine mixture. Mix well to combine using a sturdy spoon. Fold in Rice Krispies. Drop batter by tablespoonful onto prepared baking sheets to form 36 cookies. Bake for 8 to 10 minutes, or until golden brown. Remove cookies from baking sheets and cool on wire racks.

Each serving equals:

HE: 1 Fat • ¾ Bread • 13 Optional Calories

132 Calories • 4 gm Fat • 2 gm Protein • 22 gm Carbohydrate • 205 mg Sodium • 17 mg Calcium • 1 gm Fiber

DIABETIC EXCHANGES: 1 Fat • 1 Starch

If Prepared with Sugar and Butter:

200 Calories • 8 gm Fat • 2 gm Protein • 30 gm Carbohydrate

Chocolate Sugar Drops

Beautifully basic and lusciously chocolate, these sensational sweets are sure to become a lunchbox favorite at your house. Want a few extra kisses from your teenagers? Stir up a batch of these as soon as possible and see what happens! ☻ Serves 12 (2 each)

½ cup reduced-calorie margarine
½ cup SPLENDA Sugar Blend for Baking
1 egg, or equivalent in egg substitute
1 teaspoon vanilla extract

1 cup + 2 tablespoons all-purpose flour
2 tablespoons unsweetened cocoa powder
¼ teaspoon baking soda
¼ teaspoon cream of tartar
¼ teaspoon table salt

In a large bowl, combine margarine, Splenda Sugar Blend for Baking, egg, and vanilla extract using a wire whisk. In a small bowl, combine flour, cocoa powder, baking soda, cream of tartar, and salt. Add flour mixture to margarine mixture. Mix gently just to combine using a sturdy spoon. Cover and refrigerate for 15 minutes. Meanwhile, preheat oven to 350 degrees. Spray 2 baking sheets with butter-flavored cooking spray. Shape dough into 24 (1-inch) balls. Place balls on prepared baking sheets. Lightly flatten cookies with the bottom of a glass sprayed with butter-flavored cooking spray. Bake for 8 to 10 minutes, or just until firm. Do Not Overbake. Place baking sheets on wire racks and let set for 2 minutes. Remove cookies from baking sheets and continue to cool on wire racks.

HINT: Best stored in an open-air container.

Each serving equals:

HE: 1 Fat • ½ Bread • ¼ Slider • 3 Optional Calories

100 Calories • 4 gm Fat • 2 gm Protein • 14 gm Carbohydrate • 172 mg Sodium • 7 mg Calcium • 1 gm Fiber

DIABETIC EXCHANGES: 1 Starch/Carbohydrate • 1 Fat

If Prepared with Sugar and Butter:

160 Calories • 8 gm Fat • 2 gm Protein • 20 gm Carbohydrate

Date Pinwheel Cookies

If you're not a fan of dates or have never tried them, I hope this recipe will get you to reconsider—or to take a chance on these exotic and sweet fruits of a palm tree that pack so much natural sweetness inside a small package! In fact, they are so sweet I decided to pair them with smooth cream cheese and a little tart-sweet orange marmalade. ☻ Serves 8 (3 each)

¾ cup finely chopped dates
½ cup unsweetened orange juice
¾ cup SPLENDA Sugar Blend for Baking ☆
2 tablespoons + 2 teaspoons reduced-calorie margarine ☆
1½ cups + 1 tablespoon all-purpose flour ☆
1 teaspoon vanilla extract ☆
2 tablespoons fat-free cream cheese
2 tablespoons SPLENDA Brown Sugar Blend
1 egg, or equivalent in egg substitute
½ teaspoon baking soda
¼ teaspoon table salt

In a medium saucepan, combine dates, orange juice, ¼ cup Splenda Sugar Blend for Baking, 2 teaspoons margarine, and 1 tablespoon flour. Cook over medium heat for 10 minutes or until mixture thickens, stirring often. Remove from heat. Stir in ½ teaspoon vanilla extract. Set aside. In a large bowl, combine cream cheese, remaining 2 tablespoons margarine, remaining ½ cup Splenda Sugar Blend for Baking, Splenda Brown Sugar Blend, and egg until light and fluffy using a wire whisk. Add remaining ½ teaspoon vanilla extract. Add flour, baking soda, and salt. Mix gently just to combine using a sturdy spoon. Place a piece of waxed paper on counter. Place dough on waxed paper and roll into a 9-by-12-inch rectangle. Evenly spread date mixture over dough, leaving ¼-inch border at top short edge. Starting at short side, tightly roll up dough, jelly-roll style. Wrap dough in waxed paper and then in aluminum foil and freeze for at least 1 hour. Preheat oven to 350 degrees. Spray 3 baking sheets with butter-flavored cooking spray.

Unwrap dough. Using heavy thread or dental floss, cut dough into 24 (¼-inch) slices. Place slices 1 inch apart on prepared baking sheets. Bake for 10 to 12 minutes, or until light brown. Place baking sheets on wire racks and let set for 2 minutes. Remove cookies from baking sheets and continue to cool on wire racks.

Each serving equals:

HE: 1 Bread • 1 Fruit • ½ Fat • ¼ Protein • ½ Slider • 11 Optional Calories

187 Calories • 3 gm Fat • 3 gm Protein • 37 gm Carbohydrate • 196 mg Sodium • 34 mg Calcium • 2 gm Fiber

DIABETIC EXCHANGES: 1½ Starch/Carbohydrate • 1 Fruit • ½ Fat

If Preparing with Sugar, Brown Sugar, and Butter:

267 Calories • 7 gm Fat • 3 gm Protein • 48 gm Carbohydrate

Orange Marmalade Oatmeal Cookies

I'm not necessarily advocating cookies for breakfast—well, maybe brunch—but these are certainly full of morning-meal ingredients that pack a healthy punch! If you have fussy eaters who tend to skip meals or give away their lunches, you can feel good about slipping them a few of these as a snack.　　○　Serves 12 (3 each)

½ cup reduced-calorie margarine
1 egg, or equivalent in egg substitute
½ cup SPLENDA Sugar Blend for Baking
1 teaspoon lemon juice
½ cup orange marmalade spreadable fruit
1½ cups all-purpose flour
1 cup quick oats
1 teaspoon baking soda
½ teaspoon table salt
¾ cup seedless raisins

Preheat oven to 375 degrees. In a large bowl, combine margarine, egg, Splenda Sugar Blend for Baking, and lemon juice using a wire whisk. Stir in orange marmalade. In a medium bowl, combine flour, oats, baking soda, and salt. Add flour mixture to margarine mixture. Mix gently just to combine using a sturdy spoon. Fold in raisins. Drop by rounded teaspoonful onto 3 ungreased baking sheets to form 36 cookies. Bake for 8 to 12 minutes, or until golden brown. Place baking sheets on wire racks and let set for 2 minutes. Remove cookies from baking sheets and continue to cool on wire racks.

Each serving equals:

HE: 1 Bread • 1 Fruit • 1 Fat • ¼ Slider • 4 Optional Calories

193 Calories • 5 gm Fat • 3 gm Protein • 34 gm Carbohydrate • 299 mg Sodium • 14 mg Calcium • 1 gm Fiber

DIABETIC EXCHANGES: 1 Starch • 1 Fruit • 1 Fat

If Prepared with Sugar and Butter:

253 Calories • 9 gm Fat • 3 gm Protein • 40 gm Carbohydrate

James's Old-Fashioned Blondies

The ads suggest that blondes may have more fun than brunettes, and my son James believes that blondies, the good old-fashioned kind, are even more delicious than classic brownies! I guess you won't be able to make up your mind until you try these scrumptious pale bars and compare them to one of my brownie recipes. Wonder who will "win"?   ☻   Serves 12 (2 each)

¼ cup reduced-calorie
   margarine
1 egg, or equivalent in egg
   substitute
¾ cup SPLENDA Brown Sugar
   Blend
½ cup SPLENDA Sugar Blend
   for Baking

¼ cup unsweetened applesauce
1½ teaspoons vanilla extract
1½ cups all-purpose flour
1 teaspoon baking powder
¼ teaspoon baking soda
½ cup mini chocolate chips
¼ cup chopped walnuts

Preheat oven to 350 degrees. Spray a 9-by-9-inch cake pan with butter-flavored cooking spray. In a large bowl, combine margarine, egg, Splenda Brown Sugar Blend, and Splenda Sugar Blend for Baking using a wire whisk. Stir in applesauce and vanilla extract. In a small bowl, combine flour, baking powder, and baking soda. Add flour mixture to margarine mixture. Mix well to combine using a sturdy spoon. Fold in chocolate chips and walnuts. Evenly spread batter into prepared cake pan. Bake for 22 to 26 minutes, or until a toothpick inserted in the center comes out clean. Place pan on a wire rack and allow to cool completely. Cut into 24 bars.

Each serving equals:

HE: ⅔ Bread • ⅔ Fat • 1 Slider • 9 Optional Calories

182 Calories • 6 gm Fat • 3 gm Protein • 29 gm Carbohydrate • 115 mg Sodium • 36 mg Calcium • 1 gm Fiber

DIABETIC EXCHANGES: 1½ Starch/Carbohydrate • 1 Fat

If Prepared with Sugar, Brown Sugar, and Butter:

276 Calories • 12 gm Fat • 3 gm Protein • 39 gm Carbohydrate

Angie's Lemon Squares

"How about something light and lemony," my son Tommy's wonderful wife, Angie, asked on a recent visit. I was happy to oblige her with this new version of an old family favorite that is a splendid finale to a big meal. Angie, this one's for you!

☻ Serves 12 (2 each)

> 1 cup + 2 tablespoons all-purpose flour ☆
> 1¼ cups SPLENDA Sugar Blend for Baking ☆
> ½ cup reduced-calorie margarine
> 2 eggs, or equivalent in egg substitute
> ½ cup lemon juice
> ½ teaspoon baking powder
> ¼ teaspoon table salt
> 2 teaspoons grated lemon peel, optional

Preheat oven to 350 degrees. Spray a 7-by-11-inch biscuit pan with butter-flavored cooking spray. In a large bowl, combine 1 cup flour and ¼ cup Splenda Sugar Blend for Baking. Add margarine. Mix well using a pastry blender or 2 forks until mixture becomes crumbly. Pat mixture into prepared pan, building up a ¼-inch edge along sides. Bake for 12 minutes. Meanwhile, in a medium bowl, combine remaining 1 cup Splenda Sugar Blend for Baking, remaining 2 tablespoons flour, eggs, lemon juice, baking powder, salt, and lemon peel, if desired. Using an electric mixer on HIGH, beat for 3 minutes or until light and fluffy. Evenly spread mixture over partially baked crust. Continue baking for 25 to 30 minutes, or until filling is set. Place pan on a wire rack and allow to cool completely. Cut into 24 bars.

HINTS: 1. Cover your hand with a plastic bag to pat crumbs into the pan.
2. If desired, lightly dust with Grandma JO's Powdered Sugar before cutting into bars.

Each serving equals:

HE: 1 Fat • ½ Bread • ½ Slider • 5 Optional Calories

137 Calories • 5 gm Fat • 2 gm Protein • 21 gm Carbohydrate • 168 mg Sodium • 19 mg Calcium • 0 gm Fiber

DIABETIC EXCHANGES: 1 Fat • 1 Starch/Carbohydrate

If Prepared with Sugar and Butter:

213 Calories • 9 gm Fat • 2 gm Protein • 31 gm Carbohydrate

Carrot Pumpkin Bars

No, you won't turn orange if you eat more than one of these healthy but oh-so-tasty bars tonight! *Phew.* Now that we've got that fear out of the way, let's talk about the good points: Carrots and pumpkin are both packed with vitamins, but even better news is that they bring out the best in each other.   ❂   Serves 12 (3 each)

⅓ cup reduced-calorie margarine
2 eggs, or equivalent in egg substitute
1½ cups SPLENDA Brown Sugar Blend
¼ cup fat-free sour cream
2 tablespoons fat-free half & half
1 (15-ounce) can solid-pack pumpkin
1½ teaspoons pumpkin-pie spice
1½ teaspoons vanilla extract
2¼ cups reduced-fat baking mix
1 teaspoon baking powder
1½ cups finely shredded carrots
¼ cup chopped walnuts

Preheat oven to 350 degrees. Spray an 11-by-15-inch jelly-roll pan with butter-flavored cooking spray. In a large bowl, combine margarine, eggs, and Splenda Brown Sugar Blend using a wire whisk. Stir in sour cream, half & half, pumpkin, pumpkin-pie spice, and vanilla extract. In a small bowl, combine baking mix and baking powder. Add baking mix mixture to margarine mixture. Mix gently just to combine using a sturdy spoon. Fold in carrots and walnuts. Evenly spread batter into prepared pan using a rubber spatula. Bake for 20 to 25 minutes, or until a toothpick inserted in center comes out clean. Place pan on a wire rack and allow to cool completely. Cut into 36 bars.

HINT: If desired, lightly dust with Grandma JO's Powdered Sugar or frost with Grandma JO's Frosting Glaze.

Each serving equals:

HE: 1 Fat • ¾ Bread • ⅓ Protein • ⅓ Vegetable • ¾ Slider • 4 Optional Calories

232 Calories • 8 gm Fat • 4 gm Protein • 36 gm Carbohydrate • 396 mg Sodium • 86 mg Calcium • 3 gm Fiber

DIABETIC EXCHANGES: 2 Starch/Carbohydrate • 1 Fat • ½ Meat

If Prepared with Brown Sugar and Butter:

352 Calories • 16 gm Fat • 4 gm Protein • 48 gm Carbohydrate

Tom's Pumpkin Bars

I'll always deny that I found my son Tommy next to the biggest pumpkin in my pumpkin patch, but I will admit that my youngest son is *extremely* fond of pumpkin in all kinds of dishes! He's always curious to know what I will stir up next, and he knows that any dish based on pumpkin is bound to be moist and delectable.

Serves 12 (3 each)

⅓ cup reduced-calorie margarine
2 eggs, or equivalent in egg substitute
½ cup SPLENDA Sugar Blend for Baking
½ cup SPLENDA Brown Sugar Blend
1 (15-ounce) can solid-pack pumpkin
3 tablespoons fat-free sour cream
2¼ cups reduced-fat baking mix
2 teaspoons pumpkin-pie spice
1 teaspoon baking powder
¾ cup seedless raisins
½ cup chopped walnuts

Preheat oven to 350 degrees. Spray an 11-by-15-inch jelly-roll pan with butter-flavored cooking spray. In a large bowl, combine margarine, eggs, Splenda Sugar Blend for Baking, and Splenda Brown Sugar Blend using a wire whisk. Stir in pumpkin and sour cream. In a small bowl, combine baking mix, pumpkin-pie spice, and baking powder. Add baking mix mixture to margarine mixture. Mix well to combine using a sturdy spoon. Fold in raisins and walnuts. Evenly spread batter into prepared pan using a rubber spatula. Bake for 20 to 30 minutes, or until a toothpick inserted in center comes out clean. Place pan on a wire rack and allow to cool completely. Cut into 36 bars.

HINT: If desired, frost with Grandma JO's Frosting Glaze.

Each serving equals:

HE: 1 Bread • 1 Fat • ½ Fruit • ⅓ Protein • ½ Slider • 1 Optional Calorie

236 Calories • 8 gm Fat • 4 gm Protein • 37 gm Carbohydrate • 376 mg Sodium • 75 mg Calcium • 2 gm Fiber

DIABETIC EXCHANGES: 2 Starch/Carbohydrate • 1 Fat • ½ Fruit

If Prepared with Sugar, Brown Sugar, Butter, and Regular Baking Mix:

327 Calories • 15 gm Fat • 4 gm Protein • 44 gm Carbohydrate

Chocolate Oat Bars

If you've got a son or daughter serving overseas and you want to send cookies, you need to think about which treats will withstand the long journey and the jostling they may receive along the way. I recommend any of my bar cookies, especially those made with oats, which tend to be sturdy and as nutritious as they are yummy.

◒ Serves 12 (2 each)

> ½ cup reduced-calorie margarine
> ¾ cup + 1 tablespoon SPLENDA Sugar Blend for
>   Baking ☆
> 1 egg, or equivalent in egg substitute
> 2 tablespoons fat-free half & half
> 1 cup + 2 tablespoons all-purpose flour
> 1½ cups quick oats
> 2 tablespoons + 1 teaspoon unsweetened
>   cocoa powder ☆
> ½ teaspoon baking soda
> 1 teaspoon ground cinnamon

Preheat oven to 375 degrees. Spray a 7-by-11-inch biscuit pan with butter-flavored cooking spray. In a large bowl, combine margarine, ¾ cup Splenda Sugar Blend for Baking, and egg using a wire whisk. Stir in half & half. In a medium bowl, combine flour, oats, 2 tablespoons cocoa powder, and baking soda. Add flour mixture to margarine mixture. Mix gently just to combine using a sturdy spoon. Evenly spread batter into prepared pan using a rubber spatula. In a small bowl, combine remaining 1 teaspoon cocoa, remaining 1 tablespoon Splenda Sugar Blend for Baking, and cinnamon. Sprinkle mixture evenly over batter. Lightly spray top with butter-flavored cooking spray. Bake for 18 to 22 minutes. Place pan on a wire rack and allow to cool completely. Cut into 24 bars.

Each serving equals:

HE: 1 Bread • 1 Fat • ¼ Slider • 17 Optional Calories

153 Calories • 5 gm Fat • 3 gm Protein • 24 gm Carbohydrate • 153 mg Sodium • 16 mg Calcium • 2 gm Fiber

DIABETIC EXCHANGES: 1½ Starch/Carbohydrate • 1 Fat

If Prepared with Sugar and Butter:

222 Calories • 10 gm Fat • 3 gm Protein • 30 gm Carbohydrate

Chocolate Chip Lemon Bars

Now, here's a delightful partnership you don't often taste when it comes to bars and cookies—a blend of sweet chocolate and tart lemon that is hard to pass by! Coupled with some Splenda Blend, this dynamic duo dances up a dazzling storm.

● Serves 8 (2 each)

18 (2½-inch) chocolate
   graham-cracker squares,
   crushed into fine crumbs
6 tablespoons all-purpose flour
1 cup SPLENDA Sugar Blend
   for Baking ☆

⅓ cup reduced-calorie
   margarine
2 eggs, or equivalent in egg
   substitute
¼ cup lemon juice
⅓ cup mini chocolate chips

Preheat oven to 350 degrees. Spray a 9-by-9-inch cake pan with butter-flavored cooking spray. In a large bowl, combine graham-cracker crumbs and 3 tablespoons flour. Stir in ¼ cup Splenda Sugar Blend for Baking. Add margarine. Mix well using a pastry blender or 2 forks until mixture becomes crumbly. Pat mixture evenly into prepared pan. Bake for 12 minutes. Meanwhile, in a medium bowl, combine eggs and lemon juice. Add remaining ¾ cup Splenda Sugar Blend for Baking and remaining 3 tablespoons flour. Mix gently just to combine. Carefully pour filling mixture over partially baked crust. Continue baking for 10 minutes. Evenly sprinkle chocolate chips over top. Continue baking for 8 minutes, or until filling is set and chocolate chips just start to melt. Place pan on a wire rack and allow to cool completely. Cut into 16 bars.

Each serving equals:

HE: 1 Bread • 1 Fat • ¼ Protein • 1 Slider • 8 Optional Calories

204 Calories • 8 gm Fat • 3 gm Protein • 30 gm Carbohydrate • 159 mg Sodium • 12 mg Calcium • 1 gm Fiber

DIABETIC EXCHANGES: 2 Starch/Carbohydrate • 1 Fat

If Prepared with Sugar and Butter:

284 Calories • 12 gm Fat • 3 gm Protein • 41 gm Carbohydrate

Wacky Cake

Kitchen chemistry is a glorious mystery and endlessly fascinating to me. Why does bread rise? How is a bowl of wet dough transformed into crunchy cookies? And what brave cook first poked three holes into her pile of ingredients, poured three different liquids in, and ended with up with this slightly weird but wonderful cake?

○ Serves 12

> 2¼ cups all-purpose flour
> 1½ cups SPLENDA Sugar Blend for Baking
> ¼ cup unsweetened cocoa powder
> 1½ teaspoons baking soda
> ¾ teaspoon table salt
> 1½ teaspoons white distilled vinegar
> 1½ teaspoons vanilla extract
> ½ cup reduced-calorie margarine, melted
> 1½ cups cold water

Preheat oven to 325 degrees. In an ungreased 9-by-13-inch cake pan, combine flour, Splenda Sugar Blend for Baking, cocoa powder, baking soda, and salt. Make 3 holes in dry mixture. Fill one hole with vinegar, another with vanilla extract, and last with melted margarine. Pour water evenly over top. Using a sturdy mixing spoon, mix ingredients together until batter is smooth. Bake for 28 to 34 minutes, or until a toothpick inserted in center comes out clean. Place pan on a wire rack and allow to cool completely. Cut into 12 servings.

Each serving equals:

HE: 1 Bread • 1 Fat • ½ Slider • 18 Optional Calories

176 Calories • 4 gm Fat • 3 gm Protein • 32 gm Carbohydrate • 394 mg Sodium • 8 mg Calcium • 1 gm Fiber

DIABETIC EXCHANGES: 1½ Starch/Carbohydrate • 1 Fat

If Prepared with Sugar and Butter:

260 Calories • 8 gm Fat • 3 gm Protein • 44 gm Carbohydrate

Gingerbread Cake

If the only gingerbread you've ever tasted is the hard, dry kind used to craft factory-made gingerbread men, you're in for a real treat! The "real thing" is spicy and crumbly, fragrant with the scent of Grandma's kitchen (or what you imagine it might have smelled like!). Served with hot apple cider or a glass of nonfat milk, it's splendid on a crisp, fall evening. ❂ Serves 12

> ⅓ cup reduced-calorie margarine
> 1 egg, or equivalent in egg substitute
> ¼ cup SPLENDA Brown Sugar Blend
> 3 tablespoons unsweetened applesauce
> ½ cup molasses
> 1½ cups all-purpose flour
> 1 teaspoon ground ginger
> ½ teaspoon ground cinnamon
> ½ teaspoon baking powder
> ½ teaspoon baking soda

Preheat oven to 350 degrees. Spray a 9-inch round cake pan with butter-flavored cooking spray. In a large bowl, combine margarine, egg, and Splenda Brown Sugar Blend using a wire whisk. Stir in applesauce and molasses. In a small bowl, combine flour, ginger, cinnamon, baking powder, and baking soda. Add flour mixture to margarine mixture. Mix gently just to combine using a sturdy spoon. Evenly spread batter into prepared cake pan. Bake for 24 to 32 minutes, or until a toothpick inserted in center comes out clean. Place pan on a wire rack and allow to cool completely. Cut into 12 servings.

HINT: If desired, dust lightly with Grandma JO's Powdered Sugar or with Grandma JO's Butter Cream Frosting.

Each serving equals:

HE: ⅔ Bread • ⅔ Fat • ½ Slider • 10 Optional Calories

135 Calories • 3 gm Fat • 2 gm Protein • 25 gm Carbohydrate • 141 mg Sodium • 46 mg Calcium • 1 gm Fiber

DIABETIC EXCHANGES: 1 Starch/Carbohydrate • 1 Fat

If Prepared with Brown Sugar and Butter:

289 Calories • 9 gm Fat • 2 gm Protein • 29 gm Carbohydrate

Sponge Cake

Did you ever hear the one about the cook who was asked to separate six eggs, so she put three on one side of the kitchen and three on the other? I'm sure you already know that you need to crack open each egg and keep the yolks in one bowl and the whites in another. Some people use the two sides of the eggshell to gently move the yolk back and forth while letting the whites pour into a bowl. Others use their fingers, slightly spread, to hold the yolk while the white goes through. It may take practice to get it right, but don't worry—you will!   ☻   Serves 12

6 eggs, separated
½ cup unsweetened orange juice
1 teaspoon vanilla extract
1¾ cups SPLENDA Sugar Blend for Baking ☆
1¼ cups all-purpose flour
½ teaspoon cream of tartar

Preheat oven to 325 degrees. In a large bowl, beat egg yolks with an electric mixer on HIGH for 5 minutes or until eggs become thick and lemon-colored. Stir in orange juice and vanilla extract. Add 1 cup Splenda Sugar Blend for Baking. Continue beating on LOW for 1 minute. Increase to MEDIUM speed and continue beating for 5 minutes, or until mixture thickens slightly and doubles in volume. Sprinkle ¼ cup flour over yolk mixture. Fold in on LOW speed until combined. Repeat with remaining flour, ¼ cup at a time. Thoroughly wash and dry beaters. In another large bowl, beat egg whites on MEDIUM until soft peaks form. Add remaining ¾ cup Splenda Sugar Blend for Baking and cream of tartar. Continue beating on HIGH until stiff peaks form. Using a rubber spatula, fold 1 cup egg-white mixture into egg-yolk mixture. Then fold egg-yolk mixture into remaining egg-white mixture. Carefully pour mixture into an ungreased angel food cake pan. Bake on lowest rack in oven for 45 to 55 minutes, or until cake springs back when lightly touched. Invert cake in pan on funnel or bottle neck. Allow to cool completely, about 1½ hours. Gently loosen cake from pan with a table knife. Place serving plate on top of pan, invert, and gently shake cake loose. Cut into 12 servings.

Each serving equals:

HE: ½ Bread • ½ Protein • ¾ Slider • 11 Optional Calories

155 Calories • 3 gm Fat • 5 gm Protein • 27 gm Carbohydrate • 35 mg Sodium • 16 mg Calcium • 1 gm Fiber

DIABETIC EXCHANGES: 1½ Starch/Carbohydrate • ½ Meat

If Prepared with Sugar:

207 Calories • 3 gm Fat • 5 gm Protein • 40 gm Carbohydrate

Applesauce Spice Cake

Here is one of my husband's favorites—and it's likely to be a favorite of husbands everywhere! There's just something men love about this blend of fruits, nuts, and spices. Maybe it reminds them of childhood joys and a mom who baked, or maybe it's one of nature's little gifts to women: Make this, and he'll be putty in your hands! 🌀 Serves 8

¼ cup reduced-calorie margarine
1 egg, or equivalent in egg substitute
½ cup SPLENDA Sugar Blend for Baking
2 tablespoons SPLENDA Brown Sugar Blend
1 cup unsweetened applesauce
1¼ cups all-purpose flour
¼ cup graham-cracker crumbs
1 tablespoon baking powder
1 teaspoon baking soda
1½ teaspoons apple-pie spice
½ cup seedless raisins
¼ cup chopped walnuts

Preheat oven to 350 degrees. Spray a 9-by-9-inch cake pan with butter-flavored cooking spray. In a large bowl, combine margarine, egg, Splenda Sugar Blend for Baking, and Splenda Brown Sugar Blend using a wire whisk. Stir in applesauce. In a small bowl, combine flour, graham-cracker crumbs, baking powder, baking soda, and apple-pie spice. Add flour mixture to margarine mixture. Mix well to combine using a sturdy spoon. Fold in raisins and walnuts. Evenly spread batter into prepared cake pan. Bake for 40 to 50 minutes, or until a toothpick inserted in center comes out clean. Place pan on a wire rack and allow to cool completely. Cut into 8 servings.

Each serving equals:

HE: 1 Bread • 1 Fat • ¾ Fruit • ¼ Protein • ¼ Slider • 14 Optional Calories

---

214 Calories • 6 gm Fat • 4 gm Protein • 36 gm Carbohydrate • 402 mg Sodium • 112 mg Calcium • 2 gm Fiber

---

DIABETIC EXCHANGES: 1 Starch • 1 Fat • 1 Fruit

If Prepared with Sugar and Butter:

277 Calories • 9 gm Fat • 4 gm Protein • 45 mg Carbohydrate

Sour Cream Pound Cake

For a simply scrumptious cake that was just made to serve with good, strong coffee, try this creamy pound cake! If you've often thought that pound cake tastes a bit dry, you'll be delighted and amazed to taste how moist the sour cream makes this cake!

○ Serves 8

> ⅓ cup reduced-calorie margarine
> 3 eggs, or equivalent in egg substitute
> 1 cup SPLENDA Sugar Blend for Baking
> ⅔ cups fat-free sour cream
> ½ teaspoon vanilla extract
> 1½ cups all-purpose flour
> ¼ teaspoon baking powder
> ⅛ teaspoon baking soda

Preheat oven to 325 degrees. Spray a 9-by-5-inch loaf pan with butter-flavored cooking spray. In a large bowl, combine margarine, eggs, and Splenda Sugar Blend for Baking using a wire whisk. Stir in sour cream and vanilla extract. In a small bowl, combine flour, baking powder, and baking soda. Add flour mixture to margarine mixture. Mix gently to combine using a sturdy spoon. Evenly pour batter into prepared loaf pan. Bake for 50 to 60 minutes, or until a toothpick inserted in center comes out clean. Place pan on a wire rack and let set for 5 minutes. Remove cake from pan and continue to cool on wire rack. Cut into 8 servings.

Each serving equals:

HE: 1 Bread • 1 Fat • ⅓ Protein • ¾ Slider • 14 Optional Calories

218 Calories • 6 gm Fat • 6 gm Protein • 35 gm Carbohydrate • 175 mg Sodium • 49 mg Calcium • 1 gm Fiber

DIABETIC EXCHANGES: 2 Starch/Carbohydrate • 1 Fat

If Prepared with Sugar and Butter:

298 Calories • 10 gm Fat • 6 gm Protein • 46 gm Carbohydrate

Mom's Angel Food Cake

One of my mother's best-loved desserts was her angel food cake, which always (ALWAYS!) turned out beautifully light and firm. Each bite melted in your mouth, as if you were dining on the sweetest air in the world! Here's my version of her recipe, made healthier and with my love.   ☻   Serves 12

> 1 cup cake flour
> 1½ cups SPLENDA Sugar Blend for Baking ☆
> 12 egg whites
> 1½ teaspoons cream of tartar
> 1 tablespoon vanilla extract
> ½ teaspoon table salt

Preheat oven to 375 degrees. In a small bowl, combine flour and ¾ cup Splenda Sugar Blend for Baking. Mix well using a wire whisk. Place egg whites in a very large glass mixing bowl. Add cream of tartar. Beat egg whites with an electric mixer on HIGH until foamy. Add vanilla extract and salt. Continue beating until soft peaks form. Add remaining ¾ cup Splenda Sugar Blend for Baking while continuing to beat egg whites until stiff peaks form. Add the flour mixture, ½ cup at a time, folding in with a rubber spatula or wire whisk. Evenly pour batter into an ungreased angel food cake pan. Run a knife through batter to remove air bubbles. Bake on lowest rack in oven for 28 to 36 minutes, or until cake springs back when lightly touched. Do Not Overbake. Invert cake in pan on funnel or bottle neck. Allow to cool completely, about 1½ hours. Gently loosen cake from pan with a table knife. Place serving plate on top of pan, invert, and gently shake cake loose. Cut into 12 servings.

HINTS: 1. Egg whites beat best at room temperature.
2. For best results, use a large, *cool* glass bowl when beating egg whites. Run bowl under cold water and dry with a towel just before using, or place bowl in refrigerator for at least 30 minutes before using.

Each serving equals:

If Prepared with Sugar and Butter:

152 Calories • 0 gm Fat • 4 gm Protein • 34 gm Carbohydrate

Becky's Prize-Winning Banana Bread

You know how they say that the acorn doesn't fall very far from the oak? Well, my daughter Becky [children demonstrate they share the talents of their parents] is a good cook and baker herself, and this bread is inspired by her love for ripe bananas and her appreciation for easy recipes in her very busy life. ☻ Serves 8

> ¼ cup reduced-calorie margarine
> 1 egg, or equivalent in egg substitute
> ½ cup SPLENDA Sugar Blend for Baking
> ¼ cup SPLENDA Brown Sugar Blend
> 1 cup (3 medium) ripe bananas, mashed
> 1½ cups all-purpose flour
> 1½ teaspoons baking powder
> ½ teaspoon baking soda
> ¼ teaspoon table salt
> ½ teaspoon ground cinnamon
> ¼ cup chopped walnuts

Preheat oven to 350 degrees. Spray a 9-by-5-inch loaf pan with butter-flavored cooking spray. In a large bowl, combine margarine, egg, Splenda Sugar Blend for Baking, and Splenda Brown Sugar Blend using a wire whisk. Stir in bananas. In a small bowl, combine flour, baking powder, baking soda, salt, and cinnamon. Add flour mixture to margarine mixture. Mix gently just to combine using a sturdy spoon. Fold in walnuts. Evenly spread batter into prepared loaf pan. Bake for 35 to 45 minutes, or until a toothpick inserted in center comes out clean. Place loaf pan on a wire rack and let set for 10 minutes. Remove bread from pan and continue cooling on wire rack. Cut into 8 slices.

Each serving equals:

HE: 1 Bread • 1 Fat • ¾ Fruit • ¼ Protein • ½ Slider • 1 Optional Calorie

210 Calories • 6 gm Fat • 4 gm Protein • 35 gm Carbohydrate • 305 mg Sodium • 62 mg Calcium • 2 gm Fiber

DIABETIC EXCHANGES: 1 Starch • 1 Fat • 1 Fruit

If Prepared with Sugar, Brown Sugar, and Butter:

273 Calories • 9 gm Fat • 4 gm Protein • 44 gm Carbohydrate

Buttermilk Coffee Cake

When you're celebrating a birthday or graduation, why not start first thing in the morning with a delectable coffee cake that you made yourself? This one is an old-fashioned classic that recalls old-world bakeshops in cities like Vienna or Amsterdam. Mm-mm!

● Serves 12

> 2¼ cups all-purpose flour
> 1 cup SPLENDA Brown Sugar Blend
> ½ cup reduced-calorie margarine
> 2 teaspoons baking powder
> ½ teaspoon baking soda
> ½ teaspoon table salt
> 1 teaspoon ground cinnamon ☆
> 2 eggs, or equivalent in egg substitute
> 1 cup Grandma JO's Sweet Buttermilk
> ½ cup water

Preheat oven to 350 degrees. Spray a 9-by-13-inch cake pan with butter-flavored cooking spray. In a large bowl, combine flour and Splenda Brown Sugar Blend. Add margarine. Mix well using a pastry blender or 2 forks until mixture becomes crumbly. Reserve ½ cup crumb mixture. Stir baking powder, baking soda, salt, and ½ teaspoon cinnamon into remaining crumb mixture. In a small bowl, combine eggs, Grandma JO's Sweet Buttermilk, water, and ½ teaspoon cinnamon. Add egg mixture to crumb mixture. Mix gently to combine. Evenly spread batter into prepared cake pan. Sprinkle reserved crumb mixture evenly over top. Bake for 30 to 40 minutes, or until a toothpick inserted in center comes out clean. Place pan on a wire rack and let set for 5 minutes. Cut into 12 servings.

HINTS: 1. Recipe for Grandma JO's Sweet Buttermilk appears in last chapter.
2. Good served warm or cold.
3. Crumb mixture on top will "sink" into batter as it bakes.

Each serving equals:

HE: 1 Bread • 1 Fat • ¾ Slider • 1 Optional Calorie

185 Calories • 5 gm Fat • 5 gm Protein • 30 gm Carbohydrate • 343 mg Sodium • 109 mg Calcium • 1 gm Fiber

DIABETIC EXCHANGES: 2 Starch/Carbohydrate • 1 Fat

If Prepared with Brown Sugar, Butter, and Buttermilk:

258 Calories • 10 gm Fat • 5 gm Protein • 37 gm Carbohydrate

Cinnamon Pecan Muffins

Do you hate to get up in the morning? Or do your kids always roll over and go back to sleep when you wake them for school? Here's the solution, and it's a good one: splendidly fragrant muffins, warm from the oven and the best eye-opener I can think of!

○ Serves 8

¼ cup reduced-calorie margarine
1 egg, or equivalent in egg substitute
¼ cup Splenda Sugar Blend for Baking
¼ cup Splenda Brown Sugar Blend

¼ cup unsweetened applesauce
½ cup fat-free milk
1½ cups all-purpose flour
2 teaspoons baking powder
1 teaspoon ground cinnamon
½ teaspoon table salt
¼ cup chopped pecans

Preheat oven to 400 degrees. Spray 8 wells of a muffin pan with butter-flavored cooking spray or line with paper liners. In a large bowl, combine margarine, egg, Splenda Sugar Blend for Baking, and Splenda Brown Sugar Blend using a wire whisk. Stir in applesauce and milk. In a small bowl, combine flour, baking powder, cinnamon, and salt. Add flour mixture to margarine mixture. Mix gently just to combine using a sturdy spoon. Fold in pecans. Evenly spoon batter into prepared muffin wells. Bake for 14 to 18 minutes, or until a toothpick inserted in center comes out clean. Place muffin pan on a wire rack and let set for 5 minutes. Remove muffins from pan and continue cooling on wire rack.

Each serving equals:

HE: 1 Bread • 1 Fat • ½ Slider • 3 Optional Calories

178 Calories • 6 gm Fat • 4 gm Protein • 27 gm Carbohydrate • 330 mg Sodium • 95 mg Calcium • 1 gm Fiber

DIABETIC EXCHANGES: 1½ Starch/Carbohydrate • 1 Fat

If Prepared with Sugar, Brown Sugar, and Butter:

283 Calories • 15 gm Fat • 4 gm Protein • 33 mg Carbohydrate

Grandma's Cinnamon Rolls

My grandmother ran a boardinghouse many years ago, and her cinnamon rolls were legendary. Her boarders would rush to the table when these were on the menu and gobble them up as fast as she could take them out of the oven! ● Serves 12

> 1 (11-ounce) refrigerated unbaked French loaf
> ½ cup SPLENDA Sugar Blend for Baking
> ½ cup SPLENDA Brown Sugar Blend
> 1 tablespoon all-purpose flour
> 1½ teaspoons ground cinnamon

Preheat oven to 375 degrees. Spray an 11-by-15-inch jelly-roll pan with butter-flavored cooking spray. Unroll French loaf and lightly spray top with butter-flavored cooking spray. In a medium bowl, combine Splenda Sugar Blend for Baking, Splenda Brown Sugar Blend, flour, and cinnamon. Mix well to combine using a sturdy spoon. Sprinkle mixture evenly over top of French loaf. Lightly spray top again with butter-flavored cooking spray. Roll dough up in jelly-roll fashion. Using a sharp knife, cut into 12 rolls. Evenly arrange rolls in prepared pan. Cover with a clean cloth and let set for 10 minutes. Uncover. Lightly spray tops with butter-flavored cooking spray. Bake for 7 to 9 minutes, or until golden brown. Do Not Overbake. Lightly spray tops again with butter-flavored cooking spray. Remove rolls from pan and place on wire rack to cool.

HINT: If desired, spread Grandma JO's Butter Cream Frosting over
top of warm rolls.

Each serving equals:

HE: ¾ Bread • ¼ Slider • 19 Optional Calories

105 Calories • 1 gm Fat • 3 gm Protein • 21 gm Carbohydrate • 165 mg Sodium • 6 mg Calcium • 1 gm Fiber

DIABETIC EXCHANGES: 1½ Starch/Carbohydrate

If Prepared with Sugar, Brown Sugar, and Regular Sweet Yeast Dough:

185 Calories • 5 gm Fat • 3 gm Protein • 32 gm Carbohydrate

Homemade Fruitcake

Now, wait, don't turn the page just yet! I know fruitcake is often treated like a bit of a joke, but people who knock fruitcake have never tasted the sensational homemade kind! This recipe has a longer list of ingredients than many of my recipes do, but you don't make fruitcake every day—and the end result is worth it. Be inventive when it comes to choosing dried fruit, and maybe mix in some mango and papaya for a tropical version. ☻ Serves 16

⅓ cup reduced-calorie margarine
2 eggs, or equivalent in egg substitute
½ cup SPLENDA Brown Sugar Blend
½ cup unsweetened apple juice
2 tablespoons molasses
1½ cups all-purpose flour
½ teaspoon baking powder
¼ teaspoon baking soda
1 teaspoon ground cinnamon
¾ teaspoon pumpkin-pie spice
¾ cup diced mixed dried fruit
½ cup seedless raisins
8 maraschino cherries, quartered
½ cup chopped walnuts

Preheat oven to 325 degrees. Spray a 9-by-5-inch loaf pan with butter-flavored cooking spray. Line pan with waxed paper and spray waxed paper with butter-flavored cooking spray. In a large bowl, combine margarine, eggs, and Splenda Brown Sugar Blend using a wire whisk. Stir in apple juice and molasses. In a small bowl, combine flour, baking powder, baking soda, cinnamon, and pumpkin-pie spice. Add flour mixture to margarine mixture. Mix well using a sturdy spoon. Fold in mixed fruit, raisins, maraschino cherries, and walnuts. Evenly spread batter into prepared pan. Bake for 55 to 65 minutes or until a toothpick inserted in center comes out clean. Place pan on a wire rack and allow to cool completely. Remove fruitcake from pan. Wrap fruitcake in aluminum foil and refrigerate for at least 24 hours. Cut into 8 slices. Cut slices in half. Store leftovers in an airtight container.

HINT: 2 teaspoons rum extract can be added to apple-juice mixture before stirring into flour mixture.

Each serving equals:

HE: ¾ Fruit • ¾ Fat • ½ Bread • ¼ Protein • ¼ Slider • 9 Optional Calories

161 Calories • 5 gm Fat • 3 gm Protein • 26 gm Carbohydrate • 102 mg Sodium • 33 mg Calcium • 2 gm Fiber

DIABETIC EXCHANGES: 1 Fruit • 1 Fat • 1 Starch/Carbohydrate

If Prepared with Brown Sugar and Butter:

213 Calories • 9 gm Fat • 3 gm Protein • 30 gm Carbohydrate

Old-Time Lemon Meringue Pie

This diner staple is gorgeous to look at but probably unnerving to the cook who's never tried to make one from scratch! It definitely requires a little kitchen magic, some careful preparation, and more than a pinch of patience. But if you've got the courage, I've got the recipe right here.   ☽   Serves 8

> 1 refrigerated unbaked 9-inch piecrust
> 1¾ cups SPLENDA Sugar Blend for Baking ☆
> 6 tablespoons cornstarch
> ⅛ teaspoon table salt
> 1⅓ cups water
> 3 eggs, separated
> 1 tablespoon + 1 teaspoon reduced-calorie margarine
> ½ cup lemon juice
> ½ teaspoon vanilla extract
> ¼ teaspoon cream of tartar

Preheat oven to 415 degrees. Place piecrust in a 9-inch pie plate and flute edges. Prick bottom and sides with tines of a fork. Bake for 8 minutes. Place pie plate on a wire rack and allow to cool. Lower oven temperature to 350 degrees. Meanwhile, in a medium saucepan, combine 1¼ cups Splenda Sugar Blend for Baking, cornstarch, and salt. Stir in water using a wire whisk. Cook over medium heat until mixture thickens and is bubbly, stirring constantly with wire whisk. Remove from heat. In a small bowl, slightly whisk egg yolks. Gently stir in 1 cup of hot mixture using a wire whisk. Pour mixture back into saucepan. Return to heat and bring mixture to a soft boil, stirring constantly with wire whisk. Continue cooking for 2 minutes, stirring constantly. Remove from heat. Stir in margarine and lemon juice. Carefully spoon hot mixture into cooled piecrust. In a medium bowl, combine egg whites, vanilla extract, and cream of tartar. Using an electric mixer, beat on HIGH speed until mixture forms soft peaks. Add remaining ½ cup Splenda Sugar Blend for Baking. Continue beating on HIGH speed until stiff peaks form, about 4 minutes. Spread meringue mixture evenly over lemon filling, being sure to seal to edges of piecrust.

Bake for 13 to 15 minutes, or until meringue starts to turn golden brown. Place pie plate on a wire rack and let set for 1 hour. Refrigerate for at least 2 hours. Cut into 8 servings.

Each serving equals:

HE: 1 Bread • ¾ Fat • ⅓ Protein • 1¼ Sliders • 16 Optional Calories

278 Calories • 10 gm Fat • 3 gm Protein • 44 gm Carbohydrate •
186 mg Sodium • 12 mg Calcium • 1 gm Fiber

DIABETIC EXCHANGES: 3 Other Carbohydrate • 1 Fat

If Prepared with Sugar and Butter:

367 Calories • 11 gm Fat • 3 gm Protein • 64 gm Carbohydrate

Grandma JO's
Baking Secrets

I've always considered it a delicious challenge to do the culinary "impossible"—to find a way to reinvent the favorite recipes of my readers. Again and again, I've taken beloved dishes full of high-calorie elements, recipes that are high in fat and in sugar, and I've given them the "Healthy Exchanges" treatment, with delectable results. Sometimes, it's taken me many tries (and many failures) before I figured out the right combination of ingredients and preparation methods. But I don't give up. Just as a translated Japanese proverb says, "Fall down seven times, get up eight!"

I've also discovered how to make certain "store-bought" products and other delectable treats that people thought couldn't be done without a whole lot of sugar and fat, and I want to share Grandma JO's "wisdom" with you!

I'm so pleased to offer you this bonus section of Grandma JO's Baking Secrets, a scrumptious selection of recipes for toppings, sauces, frostings, fillings, and glazes, as well as amazing homemade versions of commercial products, including some dynamic dairy products that offer real help in preparing the dishes in this book.

Let me tempt you with just a few: *Grandma JO's Caramel Sauce, Grandma JO's Peanut Butter Glaze, Grandma JO's Butterscotch-Pecan Frosting, Grandma JO's Sweetened Condensed Milk, Grandma JO's South Seas Chocolate Sauce*—and so much more!

Don't you just love secrets? I do!

Grandma JO's Baked Graham-Cracker Piecrust

So what do you do if your local supermarket is out of graham-cracker piecrust and you want to make one of my recipes that calls for one? Why, you call Grandma and ask for a little advice, of course! Here's my make-it-yourself version that will definitely fit the bill.

> 1½ cups graham-cracker crumbs
> ¼ cup SPLENDA Granular
> ¼ cup reduced-calorie margarine

Preheat oven to 350 degrees. In a large bowl, combine graham-cracker crumbs and Splenda. Add margarine. Mix well using a pastry blender or 2 forks until mixture becomes crumbly. Pat crumb mixture evenly into a 9-inch pie plate. Bake for 7 to 9 minutes. Do Not Overbake. Place pie plate on a wire rack and allow to cool completely.

Based on a pie that serves 8. Each serving equals:

HE: 1 Bread • ¾ Fat • 3 Optional Calories

92 Calories • 4 gm Fat • 1 gm Protein • 13 gm Carbohydrate • 163 mg Sodium • 5 mg Calcium • 1 gm Fiber

DIABETIC EXCHANGES: 1 Starch • 1 Fat

Grandma JO's Homemade Piecrust

One of my testers nicknamed this "Make It at Midnight!" and so you can, as long as you keep these basic ingredients on hand. What a relief to know you can make a pie without racing to the store— and what an accomplishment to make any kind of pie you want in a crust you bake yourself.

1¼ cups + 2 teaspoons all-
    purpose flour ☆
1 tablespoon SPLENDA
    Granular

½ teaspoon table salt
⅓ cup cold reduced-calorie
    margarine
3 to 4 tablespoons cold water

In a large bowl, combine 1¼ cups flour, Splenda, and salt. Add margarine. Mix well using a pastry blender or 2 forks until mixture becomes crumbly. Slowly pour just enough water over crumbs until dough is moistened and just holds together. Knead dough lightly, pressing into a ball. Place a large piece of waxed paper on counter and sprinkle 1 teaspoon flour over top. Place dough on prepared waxed paper and sprinkle remaining 1 tea-spoon flour over top of dough. Place another large piece of waxed paper over dough. Gently roll into a 10-inch circle. Carefully remove top piece of waxed paper. Lay pastry crust over a 9-inch pie plate, pressing crust down into pan. Remove other piece of waxed paper. Flute edges.

HINTS: 1. Do not roll the crust too large or too thin.
        2. If using to bake pie filling in, fill with filling and bake as per recipe instructions.
        3. If using as a prebaked crust, preheat oven to 415 degrees. Prick bottom and sides with tines of a fork. Bake 9 to 11 minutes, or until lightly browned. Place pie plate on a wire rack and allow to cool completely.

Based on a pie that serves 8. Each serving equals:

HE: 1 Fat • ¾ Bread • 7 Optional Calories

104 Calories • 4 gm Fat • 2 gm Protein • 15 gm Carbohydrate • 235 mg Sodium • 5 mg Calcium • 1 gm Fiber

DIABETIC EXCHANGES: 1 Fat • 1 Starch

Grandma JO's Crumb Topping

I call this "instant dessert" because you can use it with any kind of fresh fruit to make a crunchy finishing touch. Turn an everyday meal into a feast for eyes and mouth by stirring up a batch of this!

> ½ cup + 1 tablespoon all-purpose flour
> ¼ cup SPLENDA Granular
> 3 tablespoons reduced-calorie margarine

In a medium bowl, combine flour and Splenda. Add margarine. Mix well using a pastry blender or 2 forks until coarse crumbs form. Evenly sprinkle crumb mixture over fruit filling or dessert and bake as usual.

HINT: Combine mixture just enough to make crumbs. Do not overcombine, or crumbs may turn into dough.

Based on a pie that serves 8. Each serving equals:

HE: ½ Fat • ⅓ Bread • 4 Optional Calories

50 Calories • 2 gm Fat • 1 gm Protein • 7 gm Carbohydrate • 51 mg Sodium • 2 mg Calcium • 0 gm Fiber

DIABETIC EXCHANGES: ½ Other Carbohydrate • ½ Fat

VARIATION: If desired, stir in 1 tablespoon chopped nuts just before sprinkling the topping over fruit filling.

Grandma JO's Meringue Topping

Here's a simple but spectacular way to add glamour to any pie you make—a classic meringue whose peaks will solidify your reputation as a real baker!

> 6 egg whites
> ½ cup SPLENDA Granular
> ½ teaspoon vanilla extract

Preheat oven to 350 degrees. In a large bowl, beat egg whites with an electric mixer on HIGH until soft peaks form. Add Splenda and vanilla extract. Continue beating on HIGH until stiff peaks form. Spread meringue mixture evenly over prebaked filling mixture, being sure to seal to edges of piecrust. Bake for 12 to 14 minutes, or until meringue starts to turn golden brown. Place pie plate on a wire rack and let set for 45 minutes. Refrigerate for at least 2 hours.

HINTS: 1. Egg whites beat best at room temperature.
2. Meringue pie cuts easily if you dip a sharp knife in warm water before slicing.

Based on a pie that serves 8. The meringue topping equals:

HE: ¼ Protein • 6 Optional Calories

20 Calories • 0 gm Fat • 3 gm Protein • 2 gm Carbohydrate • 42 mg Sodium • 2 mg Calcium • 0 gm Fiber

DIABETIC EXCHANGES: Free Food

VARIATION: Use coconut extract instead of vanilla extract and sprinkle 1 tablespoon flaked coconut evenly over top of meringue before baking.

Grandma JO's Powdered Sugar

For all those recipes that call for a sprinkling or even a stenciling of powdered sugar on top (think plain chocolate cake or brownies), here's my recipe for a Splenda-cized version of this baking basic.

> *1 cup SPLENDA Granular*
> *1½ teaspoons cornstarch*

In a blender container, combine Splenda and cornstarch. Cover and process on HIGH for 45 to 60 seconds, or until mixture resembles powdered sugar. Store in airtight container.

HINT: Use whenever you want a dusting of "powdered sugar" over top of dessert.

Makes ½ cup. Per each 1 tablespoon serving:

HE: 12 Optional Calories

12 Calories • 0 gm Fat • 0 gm Protein • 3 gm Carbohydrate • 0 mg Sodium • 0 mg Calcium • 0 gm Fiber

DIABETIC EXCHANGES: Free Food

Grandma JO's Heavenly Fruit Topping

I've suggested blending spreadable fruit and whipped topping for some time now, but not until this book have I named and tested it thoroughly. It's such fun to try this with different flavors of fruit spread, from blackberry to orange marmalade. If you can find it, you can make it!

¾ cup spreadable fruit (any flavor)
1 tablespoon SPLENDA Granular
¾ cup reduced-calorie whipped topping

In a medium bowl, combine spreadable fruit and Splenda. Mix gently until spreadable fruit softens. Gently fold in whipped topping. Use at once or cover and refrigerate until ready to use.

HINT: Wonderful spooned over angel food cake or pound cake.

Makes 1½ cups. Per each 3 tablespoon serving:

HE: ⅔ Fruit • 11 Optional Calories

44 Calories • 0 gm Fat • 0 gm Protein • 11 gm Carbohydrate • 0 mg Sodium • 0 mg Calcium • 0 gm Fiber

DIABETIC EXCHANGES: ½ Fruit

VARIATIONS: 1. Use blueberry spreadable fruit, ½ teaspoon coconut extract, and 2 tablespoons flaked coconut.
2. Use strawberry or raspberry spreadable fruit, ½ teaspoon almond extract, 2 to 3 drops red food coloring, and 2 tablespoons slivered almonds.
3. Use apricot spreadable fruit, ½ teaspoon vanilla extract, and 2 tablespoons chopped pecans.

Grandma JO's Buttercream Frosting

Have you sworn off frosting forever because you believe you can't risk your health or your diet? Well, I'm thrilled to give it back to you with this magnificent homemade frosting prepared the Healthy Exchanges Way. It's luscious enough to fool your husband and your kids—and to please your taste buds, too!

> ½ cup water
> 2 tablespoons nonfat dry milk powder
> 3 tablespoons all-purpose flour
> ⅓ cup reduced-calorie margarine
> 2 tablespoons fat-free sour cream
> ¾ cup SPLENDA Granular
> 1½ teaspoons vanilla extract

In a medium saucepan sprayed with butter-flavored cooking spray, combine water, dry milk powder, and flour using a wire whisk. Cook over medium heat until mixture is thick and smooth, stirring constantly. Place pan on a wire rack and let set for about 2 minutes, stirring occasionally. In a large bowl, combine margarine, sour cream, and Splenda until fluffy using a wire whisk. Add cooled flour mixture and vanilla extract. Continue mixing with wire whisk until mixture is light and fluffy.

HINTS: 1. Frosting thickens as it sets.
2. Spread over cake or bars prepared in an 8-by-8-inch baking dish or a 9-by-9-inch cake pan.

Makes 1 cup. Per each 2 tablespoon serving:

HE: 1 Fat • ¼ Slider • 7 Optional Calories

---

64 Calories • 4 gm Fat • 1 gm Protein • 6 gm Carbohydrate • 101 mg Sodium • 21 mg Calcium • 0 gm Fiber

---

DIABETIC EXCHANGES: 1½ Fat

Grandma JO's Frosting Glaze

Here's a great topping for any plain cake—coffeecake, angel food cake, or pound cake, too. It reminds me of the glaze that topped the cake doughnuts I used to devour before I started eating healthier. Now I can have frosting and not feel a single pang of guilt—and you can, too!

½ cup SPLENDA Sugar Blend for Baking
1 tablespoon + 1 teaspoon reduced-calorie margarine
3 tablespoons reduced-fat biscuit baking mix
1 tablespoon fat-free half & half
½ teaspoon vanilla extract

In a medium bowl, combine Splenda Sugar Blend for Baking and margarine. Mix well using a wire whisk. Stir in baking mix. Blend in half & half and vanilla extract using a wire whisk.

HINT: Drizzle warm glaze evenly over brownies, bars, or cakes prepared in an 8-by-8-inch baking dish or 9-by-9-inch cake pan.

Makes ½ cup. Per each 1 tablespoon:

HE: ¼ Fat • ¼ Slider • 5 Optional Calories

45 Calories • 1 gm Fat • 0 gm Protein • 9 gm Carbohydrate • 58 mg Sodium • 5 mg Calcium • 0 gm Fiber

DIABETIC EXCHANGES: ½ Other Carbohydrate

Grandma JO's
Seven Minute Frosting

I wanted you to have a great version of this classic icing that takes just about seven minutes to make. My mother was famous for it, countywide! This recipe is for a plain vanilla frosting, but you can add a bit of extract (coconut, almond, or lemon) if the spirit moves you!

> 1½ cups SPLENDA Sugar Blend for Baking
> ¼ cup cold water
> 3 egg whites
> ¼ teaspoon cream of tartar
> 1 teaspoon vanilla extract

In the top of a double boiler, combine Splenda, water, egg whites, and cream of tartar. Using an electric mixer, beat on LOW speed for 30 seconds. Place pan over bottom of double boiler filled with boiling water. Cook over medium heat, beating constantly with mixer on HIGH speed until stiff peaks form, about 7 minutes. Remove from heat. Add vanilla extract. Continue beating on HIGH for 2 to 4 minutes, or until mixture is easy to spread.

HINTS: 1. Upper part of double boiler should *not* touch water.
2. Enough to frost a cake prepared in a 9-by-13-inch cake pan or a 3-tier, 9-inch cake.

Makes 4 cups. Per each ¼ cup serving:

HE: ½ Slider • 4 Optional Calories

44 Calories • 0 gm Fat • 1 gm Protein • 10 gm Carbohydrate • 10 mg Sodium • 0 mg Calcium • 0 gm Fiber

DIABETIC EXCHANGES: ½ Other Carbohydrate

Grandma JO's
Butterscotch-Pecan Glaze

File this under "too good to be real"—but it *is* wonderfully, shockingly true and quick to fix. For a pecan lover like myself, this is the stuff that dreams are made of.

½ cup SPLENDA Sugar Blend for Baking
¾ cup SPLENDA Brown Sugar Blend
6 tablespoons reduced-fat biscuit mix
¼ cup fat-free half & half
¼ cup water
¼ cup reduced-calorie margarine
1 teaspoon vanilla extract
2 tablespoons chopped pecans

In a medium saucepan sprayed with butter-flavored cooking spray, combine Splenda Sugar Blend for Baking, Splenda Brown Sugar Blend, baking mix, half & half, water, and margarine. Cook over MEDIUM heat until mixture starts to boil, stirring constantly using a wire whisk. Continue boiling for 1 minute, stirring constantly. Remove from heat. Stir in vanilla extract and pecans. Place pan on a wire rack and let set for 5 minutes. Gently stir again just before using.

HINTS: 1. Drizzle warm glaze evenly over bars or cakes.
　　　　 2. Also good spooned over vanilla ice cream.

Makes 1½ cups. Per each 2 tablespoon serving:

HE: ½ Fat • ¾ Slider • 1 Optional Calorie

87 Calories • 3 gm Fat • 0 gm Protein • 15 gm Carbohydrate • 92 mg Sodium • 11 mg Calcium • 0 gm Fiber

DIABETIC EXCHANGES: 1 Fat • ½ Other Carbohydrate

Grandma JO's Chocolate Glaze

Easy and delicious—and CHOCOLATE! Who could ask for anything more, as the song goes? This would be great on top of a scoop of sugar- and fat-free ice cream of any flavor you can find.

> *4 teaspoons reduced-calorie margarine*
> *1 (1-ounce) unsweetened chocolate square*
> *2 tablespoons fat-free sour cream*
> *1 teaspoon vanilla extract*
> *1¼ cups SPLENDA Granular*

In a medium saucepan sprayed with butter-flavored cooking spray, melt margarine and chocolate over medium heat, stirring constantly using a wire whisk. Remove from heat. Stir in sour cream and vanilla extract. Add Splenda. Mix well to combine.

HINT: Drizzle warm glaze evenly over brownies, bars, or cakes prepared in an 8-by-8-inch baking dish or a 9-by-9-inch cake pan.

Makes ½ cup glaze. Per each 1 tablespoon serving:

HE: ¼ Fat • ¼ Slider • 17 Optional Calories

47 Calories • 3 gm Fat • 0 gm Protein • 5 gm Carbohydrate • 28 mg Sodium • 9 mg Calcium • 1 gm Fiber

DIABETIC EXCHANGES: ½ Fat

Grandma JO's Peanut Butter Glaze

For all those peanut butter lovers everywhere, here's a topping guaranteed to win your heart! We tried this on top of brownies (YUM!), over pound cake (WOW!), and even on some bar cookies before we cut them in the pan (OOH!). This one brings happiness in every bite!

> 1 tablespoon + 1 teaspoon reduced-calorie margarine
> ¼ cup reduced-fat peanut butter
> 3 tablespoons fat-free half & half
> 1 teaspoon vanilla extract
> 1 cup SPLENDA Granular

In a medium saucepan sprayed with butter-flavored cooking spray, melt margarine and peanut butter over medium heat, stirring constantly using a sturdy spoon. Remove from heat. Stir in half & half and vanilla extract. Add Splenda. Mix well to combine.

HINT: Drizzle warm glaze evenly over brownies, bars, or cakes prepared in an 8-by-8-inch baking dish or a 9-by-9-inch cake pan.

Makes ½ cup. Per each 1 tablespoon serving:

HE: ¾ Fat • ½ Protein • 15 Optional Calories

72 Calories • 4 gm Fat • 2 gm Protein • 7 gm Carbohydrate • 93 mg Sodium • 6 mg Calcium • 0 gm Fiber

DIABETIC EXCHANGES: 1 Fat • ½ Other Carbohydrate

Grandma JO's Vanilla Cook & Serve Pudding

Sometimes you can't find cook-and-serve pudding, I know that. But you may prefer to make your own because it will have fewer ingredients designed not for flavor but to preserve a commercial product on the shelves. Give this a try in any recipe that calls for cook-and-serve pudding and see if you don't think it tastes better than the original! ☺ Serves 4 (½ cup)

2 tablespoons cornstarch
½ cup SPLENDA Granular
⅔ cup nonfat dry milk powder
1¼ cups water

2 teaspoons vanilla extract
4 to 6 drops yellow food
  coloring

In a medium saucepan, combine cornstarch, Splenda, and dry milk powder. Add water. Mix well using a wire whisk. Cook over medium heat until mixture thickens and comes to a full boil, stirring constantly with wire whisk. Remove from heat. Stir in vanilla extract and yellow food coloring. Evenly spoon into 4 dessert dishes. Cover and refrigerate for at least 2 hours.

Each serving equals:

HE: ½ Fat-Free Milk • ¼ Slider • 7 Optional Calories

68 Calories • 0 gm Fat • 4 gm Protein • 13 gm Carbohydrate • 63 mg Sodium • 150 mg Calcium • 0 gm Fiber

DIABETIC EXCHANGES: ½ Fat-Free Milk

VARIATIONS: For chocolate cook & serve, add 2 tablespoons unsweetened cocoa powder when adding cornstarch, increase amount of Splenda to ¾ cup, and omit yellow food coloring.

Each serving equals:

HE: ½ Fat-Free Milk • ¼ Slider • 19 Optional Calories

88 Calories • 0 gm Fat • 5 gm Protein • 17 gm Carbohydrate • 63 mg Sodium • 153 mg Calcium • 1 gm Fiber

DIABETIC EXCHANGES: ½ Fat-Free Milk • ½ Other Carbohydrate

Grandma JO's Fruit Pie Filling

I've gotten mail from readers whose grocery stores carry only one or two flavors of pie filling—and I know how frustrating that must be for them. So here's my solution: Make whatever flavor you desire, from peach to passionfruit, pineapple to mango, and enjoy!

1 cup water
3 tablespoons cornstarch
¾ cup SPLENDA Granular
8 to 10 drops complementary food coloring, optional
2 cups peeled and chopped fruit (any kind)

In a medium saucepan, combine water, cornstarch, and Splenda using a wire whisk. Stir in food coloring. Add fruit. Mix gently just to combine using a sturdy spoon. Cook over medium heat until mixture thickens and starts to boil, stirring often, being careful not to crush fruit. Remove from heat. Place saucepan on a wire rack and allow to cool completely.

HINTS: 1. Use in any recipe that calls for a (20-ounce) can of purchased fruit pie filling.
2. Fresh fruit, frozen unsweetened fruit, or canned fruit packed in fruit juice can be used.
3. If using canned fruit packed in juice, reserve fruit liquid and use as part of water.

Makes about 2½ cups. The entire recipe equals:

HE: 2 Fruit • 163 Optional Calories

269 Calories • 0 gm Fat • 2 gm Protein • 65 gm Carbohydrate • 5 mg Sodium • 53 mg Calcium • 6 gm Fiber

DIABETIC EXCHANGES: 2 Fruit • 2 Other Carbohydrate

Grandma JO's Apple Pie Filling

Homemade apple-pie is easier than you ever imagined when you know the secret to making your own pie filling! This method produces a juicy, satisfying fruit filling that will truly amaze you with its ease.

> 1 cup unsweetened apple juice
> 1/4 cup cornstarch
> 1 cup SPLENDA Granular
> 4 cups cored, peeled, and thinly sliced cooking apples

In a medium saucepan, combine apple juice, cornstarch, and Splenda using a wire whisk. Stir in apples. Cook over medium heat until apples soften and mixture thickens, stirring often using a sturdy spoon and being careful not to mash apples. Remove from heat. Place saucepan on a wire rack and allow to cool completely.

HINTS: 1. Use in any recipe that calls for a 20-ounce can of purchased apple-pie filling.
2. If desired, stir in 1 teaspoon apple-pie spice when removing from heat.

Makes about 2½ cups. The entire recipe equals:

HE: 6 Fruit • 216 Optional Calories

576 Calories • 0 gm Fat • 0 gm Protein • 144 gm Carbohydrate • 16 mg Sodium • 48 mg Calcium • 8 gm Fiber

DIABETIC EXCHANGES: 6 Fruit • 3 Other Carbohydrate

Grandma JO's Fresh from the Patch Strawberry Sauce

If you're a strawberry fanatic with a big patch like mine, you already know that there's no such thing as too many strawberries! But even if you purchase your berries from the farmer's market or the local grocery store, you are sure to find endless uses for this vivid red sauce. Try it over pound cake or angel food cake for a dazzling dessert.

> *4 cups finely chopped fresh strawberries ☆*
> *1 teaspoon lemon juice*
> *2 tablespoons water*
> *½ cup SPLENDA Granular*

Place 3½ cups strawberries in a large bowl. Set aside. In a blender container, combine remaining ½ cup strawberries, lemon juice, water, and Splenda. Cover and process on BLEND for 20 to 30 seconds, or until mixture is smooth. Add blended strawberry mixture to chopped strawberries in bowl. Mix well to combine. Cover and refrigerate for at least 30 minutes. Gently stir again just before serving.

Makes 4 cups. Per each 1 cup serving:

HE: 1 Fruit • 12 Optional Calories

64 Calories • 0 gm Fat • 1 gm Protein • 16 gm Carbohydrate • 2 mg Sodium • 27 mg Calcium • 3 gm Fiber

DIABETIC EXCHANGES: 1 Fruit

Grandma JO's Raspberry Sauce

Fruit sauce is always good over ice cream or frozen yogurt, and raspberry is a favorite choice in fancy restaurants. Imagine peach sauce over homemade peach ice cream, or a mixed berry sauce over your favorite strawberry yogurt, and you'll get an idea of how much fun it will be to fix your own fruit sauce.

> ¼ cup diet white-grape soda pop
> ⅓ cup SPLENDA Granular
> 3 tablespoons cornstarch
> 3 cups frozen unsweetened raspberries, thawed but not
>   drained

In a medium saucepan, combine soda pop, Splenda, and cornstarch using a wire whisk. Carefully stir in undrained raspberries. Cook over medium heat for 5 to 6 minutes, or until mixture thickens and is heated through, stirring often using a sturdy spoon and being careful not to crush raspberries.

HINTS: 1. Good warm or cold.
2. Diet lemon-lime soda pop can be used instead of diet white-grape soda.
3. Frozen unsweetened blueberries, strawberries, or peaches, finely chopped, can be used instead of raspberries.

Makes 1½ cups. Per each ¼ cup serving:

HE: ½ Fruit • ¼ Slider • 1 Optional Calorie

52 Calories • 0 gm Fat • 1 gm Protein • 12 gm Carbohydrate • 2 mg Sodium • 15 mg Calcium • 4 gm Fiber

DIABETIC EXCHANGES: ½ Fruit

Grandma JO's Hot Lemon Sauce

To perk up a leftover cake or pie and give it some real pizzazz, stir up this luscious lemony topping that makes everything it touches shine brilliantly—and taste marvelously good!

⅔ cup SPLENDA Granular
2 tablespoons cornstarch
1 cup water
¼ cup lemon juice
2 tablespoons reduced-calorie margarine
⅛ teaspoon table salt
2 to 3 drops yellow food coloring

In a medium saucepan sprayed with butter-flavored cooking spray, combine Splenda, cornstarch, and water. Mix well using a wire whisk. Cook over MEDIUM heat until mixture comes to a boil, stirring constantly. Remove from heat. Place pan on a wire rack. Stir in lemon juice, margarine, and salt. Add yellow food coloring. Mix well to combine. Let set for 2 to 3 minutes. Mix well again just before serving.

HINTS: 1. Use either fresh lemon juice or the lemon juice purchased in plastic lemon bottles. Bottled lemon juice tends to be too tart for this sauce.
2. Good warm or cold.

Makes 1 full cup. Per each 2 tablespoon serving:

HE: ⅓ Fat • 16 Optional Calories

25 Calories • 1 gm Fat • 0 gm Protein • 4 gm Carbohydrate • 70 mg Sodium • 1 mg Calcium • 0 gm Fiber

DIABETIC EXCHANGES: ½ Fat

Grandma JO's Caramel Sauce

Don't wait for Sunday to enjoy a sundae when you can make your own breathtakingly good caramel topping! Use real vanilla, not the artificial kind, to make this taste like heaven on a spoon!

1½ cups SPLENDA Brown Sugar Blend
3 tablespoons all-purpose flour
⅛ teaspoon table salt
1¼ cups water
2 tablespoons reduced-calorie margarine
1 teaspoon vanilla extract

In a medium saucepan, combine Splenda Brown Sugar Blend, flour, and salt. Add water and margarine. Mix well to combine using a wire whisk. Cook over medium heat until mixture comes to a boil, stirring constantly. Continue boiling for 2 minutes, stirring constantly. Remove from heat. Stir in vanilla extract. Let set for 2 to 3 minutes. Mix well again just before serving.

HINT: Good as a dip for sliced apples or spooned over pumpkin or apple cakes.

Makes 1¼ cups. Per each 2 tablespoon serving:

HE: ¼ Fat • ¾ Slider • 17 Optional Calories

89 Calories • 1 gm Fat • 0 gm Protein • 20 gm Carbohydrate • 63 mg Sodium • 15 mg Calcium • 0 gm Fiber

DIABETIC EXCHANGES: 1 Other Carbohydrate

Grandma JO's Hot Fudge Sauce

I bet that nine out of ten ice-cream fanatics would tell you that hot fudge is their sin of choice! It's deep, dark, and luscious, and once you try it, you just never want to endure a bowl of naked ice cream again. This is astoundingly rich, considering the nutritional info listed below—but don't worry, you deserve it!

1 cup SPLENDA Sugar Blend for Baking
¼ cup unsweetened cocoa powder
1 tablespoon cornstarch
¼ cup fat-free half & half
¼ cup reduced-calorie margarine
1 teaspoon vanilla extract

In a medium saucepan sprayed with butter-flavored cooking spray, combine Splenda Sugar Blend for Baking, cocoa powder, cornstarch, half & half, and margarine. Cook over medium heat until mixture starts to boil, stirring constantly using a wire whisk. Continue boiling for 1 minute, stirring constantly. Remove from heat. Stir in vanilla extract.

HINTS: 1. Good hot or cold.
2. Spoon hot over ice cream or drizzle over cake.

Makes 1 cup. Per each 2 tablespoon serving:

HE: ½ Fat • ¾ Slider • 2 Optional Calories

95 Calories • 3 gm Fat • 1 gm Protein • 16 gm Carbohydrate • 80 mg Sodium • 12 mg Calcium • 1 gm Fiber

DIABETIC EXCHANGES: 1 Other Carbohydrate • ½ Fat

Grandma JO's Very Chocolate-Chocolate Sauce

Remember how they used to say about New York City that it was "so nice, they named it twice"? Well, this is not just chocolate sauce, this is good enough to be named twice, and *very* good to boot!

> 1 cup nonfat dry milk powder
> 1½ cups warm water
> 2 tablespoons reduced-calorie margarine
> ½ cup unsweetened cocoa powder
> ¾ cup SPLENDA Granular
> 1 tablespoon cornstarch
> 1½ teaspoons vanilla extract

In a medium saucepan sprayed with butter-flavored cooking spray, combine dry milk powder and water. Stir in margarine. Cook over medium heat until margarine melts, stirring often using a wire whisk. Add cocoa powder, Splenda, and cornstarch. Mix well to combine. Continue cooking over medium heat for 3 to 5 minutes, or until mixture thickens and is hot, stirring constantly. Remove from heat. Stir in vanilla extract.

HINT: Good served warm or cold.

Makes 1½ cups. Per each ¼ cup serving:

HE: ½ Fat-Free Milk • ½ Fat • ¼ Slider • 13 Optional Calories

95 Calories • 3 gm Fat • 4 gm Protein • 13 gm Carbohydrate • 110 mg Sodium • 161 mg Calcium • 2 gm Fiber

DIABETIC EXCHANGES: ½ Fat-Free Milk • ½ Fat

Grandma JO's South Seas Chocolate Sauce

Here's a kid-pleaser for kids of every age from 4 to 104! It's undeniably scrumptious, outrageously good, and perfect to top all kinds of cakes as well as your favorite ice creams.

2 tablespoons cornstarch
2/3 cup dry milk powder
1/4 cup unsweetened cocoa powder
3/4 cup SPLENDA Granular
1 1/2 cups water
1 teaspoon coconut extract
1/2 cup miniature marshmallows
3 tablespoons chopped pecans
3 tablespoons flaked coconut

In a medium saucepan, combine cornstarch, dry milk powder, cocoa powder, and Splenda. Add water. Mix well to combine using a wire whisk. Cook over medium heat for 6 to 8 minutes, or until mixture thickens and starts to boil, stirring constantly with a wire whisk. Remove from heat. Stir in coconut extract, marshmallows, pecans, and coconut. Serve at once.

HINTS: 1. Reheats beautifully in microwave.
2. Great spooned over sugar- and fat-free ice cream or angel food cake.

Makes 2 cups. Per each 1/4 cup serving:

HE: 1/3 Fat • 1/4 Fat-Free Milk • 1/4 Slider • 13 Optional Calories

87 Calories • 3 gm Fat • 3 gm Protein • 12 gm Carbohydrate • 39 mg Sodium • 80 mg Calcium • 1 gm Fiber

DIABETIC EXCHANGES: 1/2 Fat • 1/2 Other Carbohydrate

Grandma JO's Vanilla Crème Fraîche

This tangier, less sweet cream topping is wonderful on fruits of all kinds. If you want to offer your guests a dessert that would be at home in a fancy restaurant, try this!

> ¾ cup plain fat-free yogurt
> ⅓ cup nonfat dry milk powder
> ⅓ cup SPLENDA Granular
> 2 teaspoons vanilla extract
> ¾ cup reduced-calorie whipped topping

In a large bowl, combine yogurt, dry milk powder, and Splenda using a wire whisk. Stir in vanilla extract. Gently fold in whipped topping.

HINT: Use this as a topping for fruit and dessert.

Makes 1½ cups. Per each ¼ cup serving:

HE: ⅓ Fat-Free Milk • 10 Optional Calories

53 Calories • 1 gm Fat • 3 gm Protein • 8 gm Carbohydrate • 44 mg Sodium • 111 mg Calcium • 0 gm Fiber

DIABETIC EXCHANGES: ½ Other Carbohydrate

Grandma JO's Sweetened Condensed Milk

The canned kind available in stores is so high in sugar and fat, I knew I needed to create a healthy version for use in my recipes. Splenda makes this even better than the version I first invented quite a few years ago, and I think you'll love using it.

1⅓ cups nonfat dry milk powder
½ cup SPLENDA Granular
½ cup water

In a microwave-safe mixing bowl, combine dry milk powder and Splenda. Add water. Mix well to combine using a wire whisk. Microwave on HIGH (100% power) for 45 to 60 seconds, or until mixture is very hot but not boiling. Place bowl on counter and mix well. Let set for 5 minutes. Stir, cover, and refrigerate for at least 2 hours.

HINTS: 1. Use in any recipe that calls for a can of sweetened condensed milk.
2. This will keep for up to 2 weeks in refrigerator, if properly covered.
3. You can prepare this using Splenda Blend for Baking, but you will take the nutrients up to 720 Calories, 0 gm Fat, 32 gm Protein and 148 gm Carbohydrate.
4. If you used purchased sweetened condensed milk, the nutrients would be 1,524 Calories, 36 gm Fat, 36 gm Protein, and 264 gm Carbohydrate.

The entire recipe equals:

HE: 4 Fat-Free Milk • 44 Optional Calories

316 Calories • 0 gm Fat • 32 gm Protein • 47 gm Carbohydrate •
496 mg Sodium • 1,112 mg Calcium • 0 gm Fiber

DIABETIC EXCHANGES: 4 Fat-Free Milk

Grandma JO's Sweet Buttermilk

I first shared some special dairy recipes in my *Strong Bones* cookbook, but times have changed, and so have the recipes. This makes a splendid buttermilk for baking, it means you don't have to run to the store when you need some, and it'll never go bad in your fridge because you stir it up fresh for each recipe.

> *1 cup water*
> *⅔ cup nonfat dry milk powder*
> *1 tablespoon SPLENDA Granular*
> *1 tablespoon white distilled vinegar*

In a small bowl, combine water, dry milk powder, and Splenda using a wire whisk. Stir in vinegar. Cover and refrigerate for at least 10 minutes.

Makes 1 cup. The entire recipe equals:

HE: 2 Fat-Free Milk • 6 Optional Calories

164 Calories • 0 gm Fat • 16 gm Protein • 25 gm Carbohydrate •
250 mg Sodium • 600 mg Calcium • 0 gm Fiber

DIABETIC EXCHANGES: 2 Fat-Free Milk

Menus for the Big Events That Make Life a Joy

Family Reunion "Bake Up a Storm" Brunch

Grandma's Cinnamon Rolls
Grande Strawberry Rhubarb Crisp
Sour Cream-Raisin Spice Bread
Buttermilk Coffee Cake

Festive Holiday Cookie Exchange

Josh's Walnut Triple Chocolate Bars
Banana Blondies
Cheyanne's Fudgy Brownies
Cranberry Walnut Oatmeal Cookies

Homecoming Dessert Buffet

Candy Bar Shortcakes
Raspberry Orange Crumble
Key West Cheesecake
Decadent Fudgy Brownie Pie

PTA Bake Sale

John's Homestyle Chocolate Chip Cookies
Cappuccino Cupcakes
Apple Pie Cheesecake Bars
Mixed Berry Streusel Pie

Super Bowl Sweets "Snack 'n' Cheer" Party

Cliff's Rye Bread (with cold cuts)
Tom's Pumpkin Bars
Peanut Butter Cup Cookies
Aaron's Hot Fudge Pudding Cake

Graduation "Go for It" Get-Together

Country Carrot Cake
Chocolate Walnut Meringues
Piña Colada Custard Pie
Cherry-Almond Cobbler Criss Cross

Making Healthy Exchanges Work for You

N ow you're ready to begin a wonderful journey to better health. In the preceding pages, you've discovered the remarkable variety of good food available to you when you begin eating the Healthy Exchanges Way. You've stocked your pantry and learned many of my food preparation "secrets" that will point you on the way to delicious success.

But before I let you go, I'd like to share a few tips that I've learned while traveling toward healthier eating habits. It took me a long time to learn how to eat *smarter*. In fact, I'm still working on it. But I am getting better. For years, I could *inhale* a five-course meal in five minutes flat—and still make room for a second helping of dessert!

Now, I follow certain signposts on the road that help me stay on the right path. I hope these ideas will help point you in the right direction as well.

1. **Eat slowly** so your brain has time to catch up with your tummy. Cut and chew each bite slowly. Try putting your fork down between bites. Stop eating as soon as you feel full. Crumple your napkin and throw it on top of your plate so you don't continue to eat when you are no longer hungry.

2. **Smaller plates** may help you feel more satisfied by your food portions *and* limit the amount you can put on the plate.

3. **Watch portion size.** If you are *truly* hungry, you can always add more food to your plate once you've finished your initial serving. But remember to count the additional food accordingly.

4. **Always eat at your dining-room or kitchen table.** You deserve better than nibbling from an open refrigerator or over the sink. Make an attractive place setting, even if you're eating alone. Feed your eyes as well as your stomach. By always eating at a table, you will become much more aware of your true food intake. For some reason, many of us conveniently "forget" the food we swallow while standing over the stove or munching in the car or on the run.

5. **Avoid doing anything else while you are eating.** If you read the paper or watch television while you eat, it's easy to consume too much food without realizing it, because you are concentrating on something else besides what you're eating. Then, when you look down at your plate and see that it's empty, you wonder where all the food went and why you still feel hungry.

Day by day, as you travel the path to good health, it will become easier to make the right choices, to eat *smarter*. But don't ever fool yourself into thinking that you'll be able to put your eating habits on cruise control and forget about them. Making a commitment to eat good, healthy food and sticking to it takes some effort. But with all the good-tasting recipes in this Healthy Exchanges cookbook, just think how well you're going to eat—and enjoy it—from now on!

Healthy Lean Bon Appétit!

Index

Aaron (grandson), 187
Almonds
    Cherry Cobbler Criss Cross, 159, 306
    -Poppy Seed Bread, 35
Altitude, 5
Angel food cakes, 89–90, 95, 285, 287, 295
    Mom's, 267–68
    Roll, Cherry, 97
Angie (Tommy's wife), 251
Animal Dreams (Kingsolver), 1
Apple-pie spice, 74, 158
Apples
    Betty, Old Time, 166
    caramel sauce for, 298
    Cinnamon Cobbler, 171–72
    Cranberry Meringue Dessert, 188
    Crisp, Mom's Old-Fashioned, 167
    Crisp Pie, 204
    Fruit Baked, 165
    Johnny Appleseed Nut Bread, 74
    Pie Cheesecake Bars, 153–54, 306
    Pie Filling, Grandma JO's, 294
    Pie, Impossible French, 206
Applesauce
    Raisin Rum Cake, 118
    Spice Cake, 265
    Splenda combined with, 122
Apricots
    Chocolate Chip Cheesecake Muffins,
        67–68
    Chocolate Chip Oatmeal Cookies, 243–44
    Coconut Bars, 148
    Graham Bread, 45
    -Raisin Nut Bread, 46
Astaire, Fred, 61

Bake sale menu, 306
Baking
    as ancient art, 2–3, 19
    creativity of, 6
    as family tradition, 1, 2–3, 6–7, 78
    with Healthy Exchanges, 3–4
    high altitude, 5
    humidity and, 5, 22, 197
    during 1950's, 1
    satisfaction of, 2

Splenda Blends' impact on rising in, 238
    with sugar substitutes, 1
    variables in, 5
Baking powder, 57
    Biscuits, Grandma's, 84
Baking soda, 57
Baking tips
    for bars, 121–23
    for cakes, 87–91
    for cheesecakes, 195–200
    for coffee cakes, 56–58
    for cookies, 121–23
    for desserts, 157–58
    for muffins, 56–58
    for pies, 195–200
    for quick breads, 56–58
    for Splenda Sugar Blends, 238
    for yeast breads, 19–23
Bananas
    Bars, 149
    Blondies, 137, 305
    Blueberry Bread, 72
    Bread, Becky's Prize-Winning, 269–70
    browning of, 183
    Cake, Scrumptious, 117
    Chocolate Chip Quick Bread, 76
    Coconut Bran Bread, 50
    Cranberry Muffins, 63
    Pudding, Southern, 183–84
Barbara (friend), 6, 59, 111, 231
Barm Brack Bread, 53
Bars, 131–55. *See also* Glazes
    Angie's Lemon Squares, 251–52
    Apple Pie Cheesecake, 153–54, 306
    baking tips for, 121–23
    Banana, 149
    Carrot Pumpkin, 253–54
    Cherry Cheese, 151–52
    Chocolate Cappuccino Chip, 145
    Chocolate Cherry, 141–42
    Chocolate Chip Lemon, 259
    Chocolate Nut, 139–40
    Chocolate Oat, 257–58
    Coconut Apricot, 148
    Creamy Lime Coconut, 147
    Five Layer, 155

Bars (*continued*)
    Holiday Raisin, 150
    James's Old-Fashioned Blondies, 250
    Josh's Walnut Triple Chocolate, 143–44, 305
    Lemon Crumb, 146
    Raspberry Chocolate Chip, 138
    Tom's Pumpkin, 255–56, 306
Becky (daughter), 269
Berries. *See also specific berries*
    frozen, in muffins, 60–61
    Mixed, Streusel Pie, 203, 306
Betty, Old Time Apple, 166
Birthdays
    cakes for, 1, 99
    pies for, 209
Biscuits
    Chocolate Chip Cranberry Drop, 85
    Grandma's Baking Powder, 84
Blondies
    Banana, 137
    James's Old-Fashioned, 250
Blueberries
    Banana Bread, 72
    Crumble Pie, 201–2
    Orange Muffins, 59
Bowles, Sally, 210
Bowls, 4–5
    cleanliness of, 197
    for cookies, 121–22
Bran Coconut Banana Bread, 50
Bread machines
    cooking tips for, 19–23
    manual for, 20
    opening lid of, 23
    yeast for, 20–21
Bread Pudding, Daddy's, 161–62
Breads. *See also* Quick breads; Wheat breads;
    White breads; Yeast breads
    cream cheese in, 29
    flour, 21
    Grandma's Cinnamon Rolls, 274, 305
    for holidays, 49, 71, 77, 305
    Italian, 39–40
    quick, 55–58, 72–77
    whole-wheat v. white, 22
Brownies, 131–37. *See also* Blondies
    Cheesecake Topped Fudge, 135–36
    Cheyanne's Fudgy, 132, 305
    Chocolate Chip, 131
    Coconut Raspberry Cheesecake, 133–34
    Pie, Decadent Fudgy, 210, 305
    powdered sugar on, 284
    Walnut Pie, 209
Browning
    of bananas, 183
    of cakes, Splenda Blends' impact on, 238
    over-, of piecrusts, 196

Brunch menu, 305
Buffet menu, 305
Buffett, Jimmy, 220
Bundt cakes
    Coconut Chocolate Chip, 103–4
    Lemon Poppy Seed Coffee Cake, 81
    Orange Glow, 101–2
Buttercream Frosting, Grandma JO's, 286
Buttermilk
    Coffee Cake, 271–72, 305
    Grandma JO's Sweet, 304
    Lemon Pie, 213
    Rye Bread, 33
Butterscotch-Pecan Glaze, Grandma JO's,
    289

Cabaret (movie), 210
Cakes, 87–120. *See also* Cheesecakes; Coffee
    cakes; Cupcakes; Frostings; Glazes;
    Shortcakes, Candy Bar
    angel food, 89–90, 95, 97, 267–68, 285,
        287, 295
    Applesauce Raisin Rum, 118
    Applesauce Spice, 265
    baking tips for, 87–91
    for birthdays, 1, 99
    Black Walnut, 119
    bundt, 81, 101–2, 103–4
    Cheyanne's Fruit Cocktail, 114
    Choca-Cola, 110
    Chocolate Cream Layer, 107–8
    Chocolate Swirl, 105–6
    Chocolate Zucchini Spice, 112
    Classic Chocolate, 109
    Coconut Chocolate Chip Bundt, 103–4
    cooling, 88–90
    Country Carrot, 115, 306
    equipment for, 88–90, 100
    flour, 90
    Gingerbread, 261–62
    Island Sun, 116
    Lime Poke, 98
    Luscious Lemon Pound, 82
    Mocha Fudge, 111
    Mom's Angel Food, 267–68
    Orange Glow Bundt, 101–2
    oven temperatures and, 88–89
    Pineapple Chocolate Chip, 120
    pound, 82, 266, 285, 291, 295
    powdered sugar on, 284
    Roll, Cherry Angel Food, 97
    Roundup Time Spice, 113
    Scrumptious Banana, 117
    Sour Cream Pound, 266
    Splenda Blends' impact on browning of,
        238
    splitting into torte, 108

sponge, 89–90, 100, 263–64
Sponge, Easy, 100
Strawberry Dream, 99
testing for doneness, 89
tomato soup in, 113
toppings for, 285, 287, 291, 295, 297–301
Wacky, 260
Cakes, Pudding
    Aaron's Hot Fudge, 187, 306
    Dessert, Mocha Cappuccino, 181–82
Calcium, 17. See also specific recipes
Calories, 17. See also specific recipes
    in Splenda Granular v. blends, 238
Candy Bar Shortcakes, 193, 305
Cappuccino
    Cheesecake, 227–28
    Chocolate Chip Bars, 145
    Cupcakes, 93, 306
    Mocha Pudding Cake Dessert, 181–82
Caramel Sauce, Grandma JO's, 298
Caraway seeds, 30
Carbohydrates, 17. See also specific recipes
    in Splenda Granular v. blends, 238
Carrots
    Cake, Country, 115, 306
    Pumpkin Bars, 253–54
    and Raisin Muffins, 64
Cheese. See Cottage Cheese; Cream cheese
Cheesecakes
    Apple Pie Bars, 153–54, 306
    baking tips for, 195–200
    Brownies, Coconut Raspberry, 133–34
    Cappuccino, 227–28
    Cherry Cheese Bars, 151–52
    Chocolate Chip Mint, 231–32
    cooling/slicing, 199–200
    Easy Baked, 219
    equipment for, 196–200
    fat-free cream cheese in, 199
    Key West, 220, 305
    Latte, 229–30
    Maple Pecan, 235
    Maraschino Cherry and Chocolate, 233–34
    Muffins, Apricot Chocolate Chip, 67–68
    Pineapple Rum, 223–24
    Spectacular Raspberry, 221–22
    storing, 200
    testing for doneness, 199
    Thanksgiving Pumpkin, 225–26
    Topped Fudge Brownies, 135–36
    for weddings, 233–34
Cherries
    Almond Cobbler Criss Cross, 159, 306
    Angel Food Cake Roll, 97
    Cheese Bars, 151–52
    Chocolate Bars, 141–42
    Chocolate Dessert, 189–90

Cobbler, Classic, 175–76
Daddy's Bread Pudding, 161–62
Kuchen, 78
Maraschino, and Chocolate Cheesecake, 233–34
Upside-Down Dessert, 160
Cheyanne (granddaughter), 124
Cheyanne's recipes
    Chocolate Chip Cookies, 124
    Fruit Cocktail Cake, 114
    Fudgy Brownies, 132, 305
Choca-Cola Cake, 110
Chocolate. See also Brownies
    Aaron's Hot Fudge Pudding Cake, 187, 306
    Brownie Walnut Pie, 209
    Cake, Classic, 109
    Cappuccino Chip Bars, 145
    Cherry Bars, 141–42
    Cherry Dessert, 189–90
    Choca-Cola Cake, 110
    Cream Layer Cake, 107–8
    Daddy's Bread Pudding, 161–62
    Decadent Fudgy Brownie Pie, 210, 305
    Filling, Nut Meringue Pie with, 217–18
    Glaze, Grandma JO's, 290
    Holiday Fudge Torte, 191–92
    and Maraschino Cherry Cheesecake, 233–34
    Mocha Cappuccino Pudding Cake Dessert, 181–82
    Mocha Fudge Cake, 111
    Nut Bars, 139–40
    Oat Bars, 257–58
    Peanut Butter Chip Muffins, 65–66
    Sugar Drops, 246
    Swirl Cake, 105–6
    Walnut Meringues, 127, 306
    Zucchini Spice Cake, 112
Chocolate Chips
    Apricot Cheesecake Muffins, 67–68
    Apricot Oatmeal Cookies, 243–44
    Banana Quick Bread, 76
    Brownies, 131
    Chocolate Cappuccino Chip Bars, 145
    Coconut Bundt Cake, 103–4
    Cookies, Cheyanne's, 124
    Cookies, John's Homestyle, 241–42, 306
    Cranberry Drop Biscuits, 85
    Eggnog Muffins, 71
    Lemon Bars, 259
    Mint Cheesecake, 231–32
    Pie, 208
    Pineapple Cake, 120
    Pumpkin Holiday Quick Bread, 77
    Raspberry Bars, 138
    Raspberry Muffins, Heavenly, 61

Chocolate Sauces
  Grandma JO's Hot Fudge, 299
  Grandma JO's South Seas, 301
  Grandma JO's Very Chocolate-, 300
Cholesterol, 38, 87
Cinnamon
  Apple Cobbler, 171–72
  Pecan Muffins, 273
  Raisin Bread, Zach's, 47
  Rolls, Grandma's, 274, 305
  as substitute for other spices, 158
Cleaning up, 12
Cliff (husband), 32
Cliff's recipes
  Poppy Seed Muffins, 70
  Rye Bread, 32, 306
Cobblers
  Apple Cinnamon, 171–72
  Cherry-Almond Criss Cross, 159, 306
  Classic Cherry, 175–76
  Dessert, Rhubarb, 177
  Hawaiian Pineapple, 174
  Raspberry Pear, 173
  Strawberry Rhubarb, 178
Coconuts
  Apricot Bars, 148
  Banana Bran Bread, 50
  Chocolate Chip Bundt Cake, 103–4
  Lemon Crisp, 169–70
  Lime Bars, Creamy, 147
  Raspberry Cheesecake Brownies, 133–34
Coffee
  Cappuccino Cheesecake, 227–28
  Cappuccino Cupcakes, 93, 306
  Chocolate Cappuccino Chip Bars, 145
  Latte Cheesecake, 229–30
  Mocha Cappuccino Pudding Cake Dessert,
    181–82
  Mocha Fudge Cake, 111
Coffee cakes
  baking tips for, 56–58
  Buttermilk, 271–72, 305
  Cranberry Orange Ring, 79
  Cranberry Streusel, 80
  frosting glaze for, 287
  Lemon Poppy Seed Bundt, 81
Cola. See Choca-Cola Cake
Convenience foods, 6
Cookies, 121–55. See also Bars; Brownies
  baking tips for, 121–23
  Cheyanne's Chocolate Chip, 124
  Chocolate Chip Apricot Oatmeal, 243–44
  Chocolate Sugar Drops, 246
  Chocolate Walnut Meringues, 127, 306
  cooling/storing, 123
  Cranberry Walnut Oatmeal, 130, 305
  Date Pinwheel, 247–48

  equipment for, 121–23
  exchange menu, 305
  history of, 121
  for holidays, 150, 305
  John's Homestyle Chocolate Chip, 241–42,
    306
  Oatmeal Delite, 129
  Orange Marmalade Oatmeal, 249
  Pam's Crunchy, 245
  Peanut Butter Cup, 125, 306
  Ranger, 126
  Rolled Sugar, 239–40
  for sending overseas, 257–58
  S'More, 128
  Splenda Blends' impact on spreading of,
    238
  testing for doneness, 123
Cooking Healthy with a Man in Mind (Lund),
  7
Cooking sprays, 11
  for cakes, 88
  for cookies, 122
  flour-coating, 88
Cornmeal Bread, Sour Cream, 37
Cottage Cheese
  Bread, Herbed, 41
  Zucchini Bread, 42
Cranberries
  Apple Meringue Dessert, 188
  Banana Muffins, 63
  Chocolate Chip Drop Biscuits, 85
  Coffee Cake Orange Ring, 79
  Oatmeal Muffins, 62
  Pear Crumb Pie, 205
  Surprise Bread, 51
  Walnut Oatmeal Cookies, 130, 305
Cream cheese. See also Cheesecakes
  in breads, 29
  fat-free, 199
  on muffins, 64
  on tea sandwiches, 46
Crème Fraîche, Grandma JO's Vanilla, 302
Crisps
  Lemon Coconut, 169–70
  Mom's Old-Fashioned Apple, 167
  Pie, Apple, 204
Crumb Pie, Pear Cranberry, 205
Crumb piecrusts, 199, 280
Crumb toppings, 146, 158
  Grandma JO's, 282
Crumble, Raspberry Orange, 179, 305
Cuisinart, 42
Cupcakes
  Angel Food, 95
  Cappuccino, 93, 306
  Easy, 92
  Pretty Pink Peppermint, 94

Surprise, 96
for weddings, 87, 93
Custard pies, 197, 198
Old-Fashioned, 211
Piña Colada, 212, 306

Dairy products, fat-free, 173, 199
Date Pinwheel Cookies, 247–48
Desserts, 157–93
Aaron's Hot Fudge Pudding Cake, 187, 306
Apple Cinnamon Cobbler, 171–72
Apple Cranberry Meringue, 188
baking tips for, 157–58
buffet menu, 305
Candy Bar Shortcakes, 193, 305
Cherry Chocolate, 189–90
Cherry Upside-Down, 160
Cherry-Almond Cobbler Criss Cross, 159, 306
Classic Cherry Cobbler, 175–76
Country Baked Pudding, 163–64
Daddy's Bread Pudding, 161–62
freezing, 158
Fruit Baked Apples, 165
fruit fillings for, 158
Grande Strawberry Rhubarb Crisp, 168, 305
Hawaiian Pineapple Cobbler, 174
Holiday Fudge Torte, 191–92
for holidays, 191–92, 225–26
with ice cream/whipped topping, 158, 179, 193
Lemon Coconut Crisp, 169–70
Lemon Pound Cake Loaf, Luscious, 82
Lemon-Meringue Pudding Cups, 185–86
in microwave oven, 158
Mocha Cappuccino Pudding Cake, 181–82
Mom's Old-Fashioned Apple Crisp, 167
Old Time Apple Betty, 166
Raspberry Orange Crumble, 179, 305
Raspberry Pear Cobbler, 173
Rhubarb Cobbler, 177
Rhubarb Upside-Down, 180
saving room for, 157
Southern Banana Pudding, 183–84
Strawberry Rhubarb Cobbler, 178
topping for, 302
Diabetes, 87, 198
Diabetic Exchanges, 17. See also specific recipes
bread machines and, 20
Dickinson, Emily, 7
Diets, 3
Dill Onion Rye Bread, 44

Eating habits, healthy, 307–8
Eggnog Chocolate Chip Muffins, 71
Eggs. See also Meringues
beating, 90, 197

Bread, 25
in cakes, 90, 100
high altitude baking and, 5
limiting consumption of, 18
meringues and, 197
at room temperature, 90, 183, 186, 188
separating, 100, 263
Equipment, 4–5, 11. See also specific equipment
for cakes, 88–90, 100
cleanliness of, 197
for cookies, 121–23
measuring, 87–88
muffin pans, preventing warping of, 58, 92
for pies/cheesecakes, 196–200

Family reunion menu, 305
Fat, 17. See also specific recipes
Fat-free dairy products, 173, 199
Fiber, 17. See also specific recipes
Flour
all-purpose v. cake, 90
bread, 21
-coating cooking spray, 88
freezing, 21
gluten in, 56
measuring, 22
Focaccia Bread, 39
Food funnies, 195
Freezing
breads/muffins, 20, 57, 62
desserts, 158
pies, 198–99
recipes, 18
yeasts/flour, 21
Freud, Sigmund, 193
Frostings. See also Glazes
Buttercream, Grandma JO's, 286
Glaze, Grandma JO's, 287
Seven Minute, Grandma JO's, 288
Fruit. See specific fruit
Fruit breads, Quick
Banana Chocolate Chip, 76
Blueberry Banana, 72
Cherry Kuchen, 78
Chocolate Chip Cranberry Drop Biscuits, 85
Johnny Appleseed Nut Bread, 74
Pecan Pear Scones, 83
Zucchini Raisin Nut, 75
Fruit breads, yeast
Apricot Graham, 45
Apricot-Raisin Nut, 46
Barm Brack Bread, 53
Coconut Banana Bran, 50
Cranberry Surprise, 51
Tropical Pineapple, 52

Fruit, cakes with
  Applesauce Spice, 265
  Cherry Angel Food Cake Roll, 97
  Cheyanne's Fruit Cocktail Cake, 114
  Island Sun, 116
  Orange Glow Bundt, 101–2
  Pineapple Chocolate Chip, 120
  Scrumptious Banana, 117
  Strawberry Dream, 99
Fruit, cheesecakes with
  Key West, 220, 305
  Maraschino Cherry and Chocolate, 233–34
  Pineapple Rum, 223–24
  Spectacular Raspberry, 221–22
Fruit coffee cakes
  Cranberry Orange Ring, 79
  Cranberry Streusel, 80
  Lemon Poppy Seed Bundt, 81
Fruit, cookies/bars with
  Angie's Lemon Squares, 251–52
  Apple Pie Cheesecake, 153–54, 306
  Banana, 149
  Cherry Cheese, 151–52
  Chocolate Cherry, 141–42
  Chocolate Chip Apricot Oatmeal, 243–44
  Chocolate Chip Lemon, 259
  Coconut Apricot, 148
  Coconut Raspberry Cheesecake Brownies,
    133–34
  Cranberry Walnut Oatmeal Cookies, 130, 305
  Creamy Lime Coconut, 147
  Date Pinwheel, 247–48
  Holiday Raisin, 150
  Lemon Crumb, 146
  Raspberry Chocolate Chip, 138
Fruit desserts, 158
  Apple Cinnamon Cobbler, 171–72
  Apple Cranberry Meringue, 188
  Candy Bar Shortcakes, 193, 305
  Cherry Chocolate, 189–90
  Cherry Upside-Down, 160
  Cherry-Almond Cobbler Criss Cross, 159, 306
  Classic Cherry Cobbler, 175–76
  Daddy's Bread Pudding, 161–62
  Fruit Baked Apples, 165
  Grande Strawberry Rhubarb Crisp, 168,
    305
  Hawaiian Pineapple Cobbler, 174
  Lemon Coconut Crisp, 169–70
  Lemon-Meringue Pudding Cups, 185–86
  Mom's Old-Fashioned Apple Crisp, 167
  Old Time Apple Betty, 166
  Raspberry Orange Crumble, 179, 305
  Raspberry Pear Cobbler, 173
  Rhubarb Cobbler, 177
  Rhubarb Upside-Down, 180

  Southern Banana Pudding, 183–84
  Strawberry Rhubarb Cobbler, 178
Fruit Fresh, 183
Fruit muffins
  Apricot Chocolate Chip Cheesecake, 67–68
  Banana Cranberry, 63
  Blueberry Orange, 59
  Heavenly Raspberry Chocolate Chip, 61
  Oatmeal Cranberry, 62
  Raspberry, 60
Fruit pies
  Apple Crisp, 204
  Blueberry Crumble, 201–2
  fillings, 293–94
  Impossible French Apple, 206
  Lemon "Buttermilk," 213
  Mixed Berry Streusel, 203, 306
  Old-Time Lemon Meringue, 277–78
  Pear Cranberry Crumb, 205
  Rhubarb Raspberry Meringue, 215–16
  tips for, 197–99
Fruit sauces
  Grandma JO's Fresh from the Patch
    Strawberry, 295
  Grandma JO's Hot Lemon, 297
  Grandma JO's Raspberry, 296
Fruit, spreadable, 285
Fruit Toppings, 302
  Grandma JO's Heavenly, 285
Fruitcake, Homemade, 275–76
Fudge
  Brownie Pie, Decadent, 210, 305
  Brownies, Cheesecake Topped, 135–36
  Brownies, Cheyanne's, 132, 305
  Cake, Mocha, 111
  Pudding Cake, Aaron's Hot, 187, 306
  Sauce, Grandma JO's Hot, 299
  Torte, Holiday, 191–92

Gingerbread Cake, 261–62
Glazes
  Butterscotch-Pecan, Grandma JO's, 289
  Chocolate, Grandma JO's, 290
  Frosting, Grandma JO's, 287
  Peanut Butter, Grandma JO's, 291
Graduation menu, 306
Graham Apricot Bread, 45
Graham crackers
  crushing, 222
  Piecrust, Grandma JO's Baked, 280
Grandma JO recipes, 18, 279–304
  Apple Pie Filling, 294
  Baked Graham Cracker Piecrust, 280
  Buttercream Frosting, 286
  Butterscotch-Pecan Glaze, 289
  Caramel Sauce, 298

Chocolate Glaze, 290
Crumb Topping, 282
Fresh from the Patch Strawberry Sauce, 295
Frosting Glaze, 287
Fruit Pie Filling, 293
Heavenly Fruit Topping, 285
Homemade Piecrust, 281
Hot Fudge Sauce, 299
Hot Lemon Sauce, 297
Meringue Topping, 283
Peanut Butter Glazes, 291
Powdered Sugar, 284
Raspberry Sauce, 296
Seven Minute Frosting, 288
South Seas Chocolate Sauce, 301
Sweet Buttermilk, 304
Sweetened Condensed Milk, 303
Vanilla Cook & Serve Pudding, 292
Vanilla Crème Fraîche, 302
Very Chocolate-Chocolate Sauce, 300

Handy, Jack, 195
Healthy Exchanges. *See also specific recipes*
    baking with, 3–4
    books with, 7
    contact information for, 309–10
    explanation of, 7
    making it work for you, 307–8
    nutritional analysis, 17–18
    reinventing recipes with, 279
    Web site, 309
The Healthy Exchanges Food Newsletter, 310
Heart issues, 198
Herbs
    fresh v. dried, 43
    Herbed Cottage Cheese Bread, 41
    Onion Dill Rye Bread, 44
    Rosemary Sour Cream Whole Wheat Bread, 43
Holiday breads
    Chocolate Chip Eggnog Muffins, 71
    Pumpkin Chocolate Chip Quick Bread, 77
    Sour Cream-Raisin Spice, 49, 305
Holidays
    cookies for, 150, 305
    desserts for, 191–92, 225–26
Humidity, 5, 22, 197

Ice cream
    desserts with, 158, 179, 193
    toppings for, 289–90, 296, 298–301
Ingredients
    advance preparation of, 11–12, 21–22, 196
    division of, 18
    doubling/tripling/halving, 12–13

freshness of, 21, 57
for fruit desserts, 158
measuring, 4, 12, 22, 87–88, 158
at room temperature, 21–22, 90, 122, 183, 186, 188
from Splenda pantry, 9–10
Ireland, 2, 53
Italian breads
    Focaccia, 39
    Pimiento Italian, 40

James (son), 78, 189, 250
Japanese proverb, 279
JoAnna's Kitchen Miracles (Lund), 19
John (son-in-law), 241
Josh (grandson), 143

Kingsolver, Barbara, 1
Kitchen chemistry, 260
Kitchen timers, 12, 199
Kuchen, Cherry, 78

Latte Cheesecake, 229–30
Lebowitz, Fran, 6
Lemons, 70
    "Buttermilk" Pie, 213
    Chocolate Chip Bars, 259
    Coconut Crisp, 169–70
    Crumb Bars, 146
    Meringue Pie, Old-Time, 277–78
    -Meringue Pudding Cups, 185–86
    Poppy Seed Bundt Coffee Cake, 81
    Sauce, Grandma JO's Hot, 297
    Squares, Angie's, 251–52
Lime
    Coconut Bars, Creamy, 147
    Key West Cheesecake, 220, 305
    Poke Cake, 98
Lund, JoAnna M.
    books by, 7, 19, 304
    contact information for, 309

Maple
    Oatmeal Pie, 214
    Pecan Cheesecake, 235
Marmalade Oatmeal Cookies, Orange, 249
McNeil Nutritionals, 237
Menus, 305–6
    Family Reunion "Bake Up a Storm" Brunch, 305
    Festive Holiday Cookie Exchange, 305
    Graduation "Go for It" Get-Together, 306
    Homecoming Dessert Buffet, 305
    PTA Bake Sale, 306
    Super Bowl Sweets "Snack 'n' Cheer" Party, 306

Meringues
    Chocolate Walnut, 127, 306
    Dessert, Apple Cranberry, 188
    eggs and, 197
    humidity impact on, 197
    Lemon Pudding Cups, 185–86
    Nut Pie, with Chocolate Filling, 217–18
    Pie, Old-Time Lemon, 277–78
    Pie, Rhubarb Raspberry, 215–16
    pies, 197–98, 215–18, 277–78
    tips for, 197–98
    Topping, Grandma JO's, 283
Microwave ovens
    desserts in, 158
    reheating in, 58
Milk, Grandma JO's Sweetened Condensed,
    303
Minnelli, Liza, 210
Mint Chocolate Chip Cheesecake, 231–32
Mocha. *See* Chocolate
Muffins, 55–71
    Apricot Chocolate Chip Cheesecake, 67–68
    baking tips for, 56–58
    Banana Cranberry, 63
    Blueberry Orange, 59
    Carrot and Raisin, 64
    Chocolate Chip Eggnog, 71
    Chocolate Peanut Butter Chip, 65–66
    Cinnamon Pecan, 273
    Cliff's Poppy Seed, 70
    frozen berries in, 60–61
    Oatmeal Cranberry, 62
    oven temperatures for quick breads v., 56
    pans, preventing warping of, 58, 92
    Pirate's Pleasure, 69
    Raspberry, 60
    Raspberry Chocolate Chip, Heavenly, 61
    storing/freezing, 57, 62

Nutritional analysis. *See also specific nutrients*
    Healthy Exchanges, 17–18
    for sweetened condensed milk, 303
Nuts. *See also* Peanut Butter; *specific nuts*
    Almond-Poppy Seed Bread, 35
    Apricot-Raisin Nut Bread, 46
    Black Walnut Cake, 119
    Cherry-Almond Cobbler Criss Cross, 159,
        306
    Chocolate Bars, 139–40
    Chocolate Walnut Meringues, 127, 306
    Cinnamon Pecan Muffins, 273
    Cranberry Walnut Oatmeal Cookies, 130, 305
    Grandma JO's Butterscotch-Pecan Glaze, 289
    Johnny Appleseed Nut Bread, 74
    Josh's Walnut Triple Chocolate Bars,
        143–44, 305

Maple Pecan Cheesecake, 235
Meringue Pie, with Chocolate Filling, 217–18
Oatmeal Walnut Bread, 34
Pecan Pear Scones, 83
Walnut Whole Wheat Bread, 29
Zucchini Raisin Nut Bread, 75

Oat bran cereal, 50
Oatmeal
    Chocolate Bars, 257–58
    Chocolate Chip Apricot Cookies, 243–44
    Cranberry Muffins, 62
    Cranberry Walnut Cookies, 130, 305
    Delite Cookies, 129
    Maple Pie, 214
    Sour Cream Bread, 38
    Walnut Bread, 34
Olive oil, 39
Olsen Twins, 211
Onion Dill Rye Bread, 44
The Open Road Cookbook (Lund), 7
Oranges
    Blueberry Muffins, 59
    Cranberry Coffee Cake Ring, 79
    Glow Bundt Cake, 101–2
    Marmalade Oatmeal Cookies, 249
    Raspberry Crumble, 179, 305
Oven temperatures
    cakes and, 88–89
    for muffins v. quick breads, 56
    variables in, 5, 57, 89
Ovens
    microwave, 58, 158
    preheating, 57–58, 88–89, 158, 196
    toaster, 55

Pam (daughter-in-law), 245
Pantry, Baking with Splenda, 9–10
Peanut Butter
    Chip Chocolate Muffins, 65–66
    Cup Cookies, 125, 306
    Glaze, Grandma JO's, 291
    Quick Bread, Mom's, 73
Pears
    Cranberry Crumb Pie, 205
    Pecan Scones, 83
    Raspberry Cobbler, 173
Pecans
    Butterscotch Glaze, Grandma JO's, 289
    Cinnamon Muffins, 273
    Maple Cheesecake, 235
    Pear Scones, 83
Peppermint Cupcakes, Pretty Pink, 94
Phyllis (recipe tester), 129
Piecrusts
    crumb, 199, 280

double, 197
Graham Cracker, Grandma JO's Baked, 280
Homemade, Grandma JO's, 281
over-browning, 196
refrigerated, 196
soggy, 196
tips for, 196–97, 199
Pies, 195–235. *See also* Cheesecakes
Apple, Cheesecake Bars, 153–54, 306
Apple Crisp, 204
Apple, Impossible French, 206
baking tips for, 195–200
birds, 197
for birthdays, 209
Blueberry Crumble, 201–2
Brownie Walnut, 209
Chocolate Chip, 208
cooling, 196, 198–200
custard, 197, 198, 211–12, 306
cutting/serving, 198–200
Decadent Fudgy Brownie, 210, 305
equipment for, 196–200
Filling, Grandma JO's Apple, 294
Filling, Grandma JO's Fruit, 293
freezing, 198–99
fruit, 197–99, 201–6, 215–16
Grandma's Old-Fashioned Pumpkin, 207
heaven, 195
Lemon "Buttermilk," 213
meringue, 197–98, 215–18, 277–78
Mixed Berry Streusel, 203, 306
Nut Meringue, with Chocolate Filling, 217–18
Oatmeal Maple, 214
Old-Fashioned Custard, 211
Old-Time Lemon Meringue, 277–78
Pear Cranberry Crumb, 205
Piña Colada Custard, 212, 306
Rhubarb Raspberry Meringue, 215–16
storing, 198–200
testing for doneness, 197, 199
thawing, 199
topping for, 297
Pimiento Italian Bread, 40
Piña Colada Custard Pie, 212, 306
Pineapple
Bread, Tropical, 52
Chocolate Chip Cake, 120
Cobbler, Hawaiian, 174
Rum Cheesecake, 223–24
Plate size, 308
Poppy Seeds
-Almond Bread, 35
Lemon Bundt Coffee Cake, 81
Muffins, Cliff's, 70
Portion size, 308

Pound cakes
Luscious Lemon, 82
Sour Cream, 266
toppings for, 285, 291, 295
Powdered Sugar, Grandma JO's, 284
Products, recommended, 9–10
Protein, 17. *See also specific recipes*
Pudding Cakes
Aaron's Hot Fudge, 187, 306
Dessert, Mocha Cappuccino, 181–82
Puddings
Bread, Daddy's, 161–62
Country Baked, 163–64
Cups, Lemon-Meringue, 185–86
Southern Banana, 183–84
substitutions with, 12
Vanilla Cook & Serve, Grandma JO's, 292
Pumpkin-pie spice, 12, 158
Pumpkins
Bars, Tom's, 255–56, 306
Carrot Bars, 253–54
Cheesecake, Thanksgiving, 225–26
Chocolate Chip Holiday Quick Bread, 77
Pie, Grandma's Old-Fashioned, 207

Quick breads, 55–58, 72–77. *See also* Biscuits;
Coffee cakes
baking tips for, 56–58
Banana Chocolate Chip, 76
Becky's Prize-Winning Banana, 269–70
Blueberry Banana, 72
Cherry Kuchen, 78
Johnny Appleseed Nut Bread, 74
Lemon Pound Cake Loaf, Luscious, 82
Mom's Peanut Butter, 73
oven temperatures for muffins v., 56
Pecan Pear Scones, 83
Pumpkin Chocolate Chip Holiday, 77
storing/freezing, 57
Zucchini Raisin Nut, 75

Raisins
Applesauce Rum Cake, 118
Apricot Nut Bread, 46
Bars, Holiday, 150
and Carrot Muffins, 64
Cinnamon Bread, Zach's, 47
Nut Zucchini Bread, 75
Sour Cream Spice Bread, 49, 305
Sunshine Bread, 48
Raspberries
Cheesecake, Spectacular, 221–22
Chocolate Chip Bars, 138
Chocolate Chip Muffins, Heavenly, 61
Coconut Cheesecake Brownies, 133–34
Muffins, 60

Raspberries (*continued*)
  Orange Crumble, 179, 305
  Pear Cobbler, 173
  Rhubarb Meringue Pie, 215–16
  Sauce, Grandma JO's, 296
Recipes
  changes with Splenda, 19
  converting to Splenda Sugar Blends, 238
  doubling/tripling/halving, 12–13
  freezing, 18
  rating/comments on, 13, 23
  reading/following, 11, 12
  reinventing readers', 279
Rhubarb
  Cobbler Dessert, 177
  Raspberry Meringue Pie, 215–16
  Strawberry Cobbler, 178
  Strawberry Crisp, Grande, 168, 305
  Upside-Down Dessert, 180
Rice Krispies, 245
Rogers, Ginger, 61
Room temperature
  eggs at, 90, 183, 186, 188
  ingredients at, 21–22, 122
  refrigerated piecrusts at, 196
  storing pies at, 198
Rosemary Sour Cream Whole Wheat Bread,
    43
Rum
  Applesauce Raisin Cake, 118
  Pineapple Cheesecake, 223–24
Rye breads
  "Buttermilk," 33
  Cliff's, 32, 306
  Light, 30
  Onion Dill, 44
  Swedish, 31

Salt, 22. *See also* Sodium
Saturday Night Live (TV show), 195
Sauces. *See also* Applesauce
  Caramel, Grandma JO's, 298
  chocolate, 299–301
  Lemon, Grandma JO's Hot, 297
  Raspberry, Grandma JO's, 296
  Strawberry, Grandma JO's Fresh from the
    Patch, 295
Scones, Pecan Pear, 83
Seeds
  caraway, 30
  poppy, 35, 70, 81
Shortcakes, Candy Bar, 193, 305
Soda pop
  Choca-Cola Cake, 110
  Lemon-Meringue Pudding Cups, 185–86
Sodium, 17. *See also specific recipes*

Soup, tomato, 113
Sour cream, 173
  Cornmeal Bread, 37
  Oatmeal Bread, 38
  Pound Cake, 266
  -Raisin Spice Bread, 49, 305
  Rosemary Whole Wheat Bread, 43
Spatulas, 4–5
Spices. *See also* Cinnamon
  apple-pie, 74, 158
  Cake, Applesauce, 265
  Cake, Chocolate Zucchini, 112
  Cake, Roundup Time, 113
  doubling, 12–13
  pumpkin-pie, 12, 158
  Sour Cream-Raisin Bread, 49, 305
  substituting, 158
Splenda
  aftertaste from, 237
  applesauce combined with, 122
  FDA approval for, 237
  Granular, 238
  margarine combined with, 90–91, 122
  meringues and, 197
  Pantry, Baking with, 9–10
  reasons for using, 1
  recipe changes with, 19
  sugar v., 238
  website, 237
Splenda Sugar Blends for Baking, 237–78
  baking tips for, 238
  breads with, 269–70
  brown sugar, 237–38
  cakes with, 260–68
  cinnamon rolls with, 274
  coffee cake with, 271–72
  cookies/bars with, 239–59
  fruitcake with, 275–76
  muffins with, 273
  pie with, 277–78
  recipe conversion to, 238
  sweetened condensed milk with, 303
Sponge cakes, 89–90, 100, 263–64
St. Brigid's Feast Day, 53
Strawberries
  Dream Cake, 99
  Rhubarb Cobbler, 178
  Rhubarb Crisp, Grande, 168, 305
  Sauce, Grandma JO's Fresh from the Patch,
    295
Streusel
  Coffee Cake, Cranberry, 80
  Pie, Mixed Berry, 203, 306
The Strong Bones Healthy Exchanges Cookbook
    (Lund), 304
Substitutions. *See also* Splenda

with puddings, 12
with spices, 158
sugar, 1
Sugar
brown, 237–38
Cookies, Rolled, 239–40
Drops, Chocolate, 246
Powdered, Grandma JO's, 284
Splenda v., 238
Sugar Blends. *See* Splenda Sugar Blends for Baking
Sugar substitutes, 1. *See also* Splenda
Sunshine Bread, 48
Super Bowl menu, 306
Sweet Potato Bread, 36
Sweetened Condensed Milk, Grandma JO's, 303

Temperatures
oven, 5, 56, 57, 88–89, 89
room, 21–22, 90, 122, 183, 186, 188, 196, 198
Ten Commandments of Successful Cooking, 11–13
Toaster ovens, 55
Tomato soup, in cake, 113
Tommy (son), 251, 255
Toppings. *See also* Whipped topping
for cakes, 285, 287, 291, 295, 297–301
crumb, 146, 158, 282
fruit, 285, 302
Meringue, Grandma JO's, 283
for pies, 297
Tortes
cakes split into, 108
Holiday Fudge, 191–92

Upside-Down Desserts
Cherry, 160
Rhubarb, 180

Vanilla
Cook & Serve Pudding, 292
Crème Fraîche, Grandma JO's, 302
Vegetables. *See also specific vegetables*
Carrot and Raisin Muffins, 64
Carrot Cake, Country, 115, 306
Carrot Pumpkin Bars, 253–54
Onion Dill Rye Bread, 44
Pumpkin Bars, Tom's, 255–56, 306
Pumpkin Cheesecake, Thanksgiving, 225–26
Pumpkin Chocolate Chip Holiday Quick Bread, 77
Pumpkin Pie, Grandma's Old-Fashioned, 207

Sweet Potato Bread, 36
Zucchini Cottage Cheese Bread, 42
Zucchini Spice Cake, Chocolate, 112

Walnuts
Brownie Pie, 209
Cake, Black, 119
Chocolate Meringues, 127, 306
Cranberry Oatmeal Cookies, 130, 305
Oatmeal Bread, 34
Triple Chocolate Bars, Josh's, 143–44, 305
Whole Wheat Bread, 29
Watts, Colin, 237
websites
Healthy Exchanges, 309
Splenda, 237
Weddings
cheesecakes for, 233–34
cupcakes for, 87, 93
Weight loss, 7, 198
nutritional analysis for, 17
Wheat breads
Basic Whole Wheat, 26
Maple Wheat, 27
Rosemary Sour Cream Whole Wheat, 43
Walnut Whole Wheat, 29
white v., 22
Whole Wheat Molasses, 28
Whipped topping. *See also specific recipes*
on cheesecakes, 199
desserts with ice cream or, 158, 179, 193
spreadable fruit and, 285
White breads
"Homemade," 24
whole wheat v., 22

Yeast breads, 19–53
Almond-Poppy Seed, 35
Apricot Graham, 45
Apricot-Raisin Nut, 46
baking tips for, 19–23
Barm Brack, 53
Basic Whole Wheat, 26
"Buttermilk" Rye, 33
Cliff's Rye, 32, 306
Coconut Banana Bran, 50
Cranberry Surprise, 51
Egg, 25
Focaccia, 39
freezing, 20
Herbed Cottage Cheese, 41
"Homemade" white, 24
Light Rye, 30
Maple Wheat, 27
Oatmeal Sour Cream, 38

Yeast breads (*continued*)
  Oatmeal Walnut, 34
  Onion Dill Rye, 44
  Pimiento Italian, 40
  Rosemary Sour Cream Whole Wheat, 43
  Sour Cream Cornmeal, 37
  Sour Cream-Raisin Spice, 49, 305
  Sunshine, 48
  Swedish Rye, 31
  Sweet Potato, 36
  thawing, 20
  Tropical Pineapple, 52
  Walnut Whole Wheat, 29

  Whole Wheat Molasses, 28
  Zach's Cinnamon Raisin, 47
  Zucchini Cottage Cheese, 42
Yeasts
  bread machine v. regular, 20–21
  freezing, 21
Yogurt, frozen, 296

Zach (grandson), 47
Zach's Cinnamon Raisin Bread, 47
Zucchini
  Chocolate Spice Cake, 112
  Cottage Cheese Bread, 42
  Raisin Nut Bread, 75

I Want to Hear from You...

Besides my family, the love of my life is creating "common folk" healthy recipes and solving everyday cooking questions in The Healthy Exchanges Way. Everyone who uses my recipes is considered part of the Healthy Exchanges Family, so please write to me if you have any questions, comments, or suggestions. I will do my best to answer. With your support, I'll continue to stir up even more recipes and cooking tips for the family in the years to come.

Write to: JoAnna M. Lund
            c/o Healthy Exchanges, Inc.
            P.O. Box 80
            DeWitt, IA 52742-0080

If you prefer, you can fax me at 1-563-659-2126 or contact me via e-mail by writing to HealthyJo@aol.com. Or visit my Healthy Exchanges website at: http: www.healthyexchanges.com.

Now That You've Seen *Baking Healthy with Splenda*, Why Not Order *The Healthy Exchanges Food Newsletter?*

If you enjoyed the recipes in this cookbook and would like to cook up even more of my "common folk" healthy dishes, you may want to subscribe to *The Healthy Exchanges Food Newsletter.*

This monthly 12-page newsletter contains 30-plus new recipes *every month* in such columns as:

- Reader Exchange
- Reader Requests
- Recipe Makeover
- Micro Corner
- Dinner for Two
- Crock Pot Luck
- Meatless Main Dishes
- Rise & Shine
- Our Small World
- Brown Bagging It
- Snack Attack
- Side Dishes
- Main Dishes
- Desserts

In addition to all the recipes, other regular features include:

- The Editor's Motivational Corner
- Dining Out Question & Answer
- Cooking Question & Answer
- New Product Alert
- Success Profiles of Winners in the Losing Game
- Exercise Advice from a Cardiac Rehab Specialist
- Nutrition Advice from a Registered Dietitian
- Positive Thought for the Month

The cost for a one-year (12-issue) subscription is $25. To order, call our toll-free number and pay with any major credit card—or send a check to the address on page 321 of this book.

1-800-766-8961 for Customer Orders
1-563-659-8234 for Customer Service

Thank you for your order, and for choosing to become a part of the Healthy Exchanges Family!